# Weight Watchers Freestyle Cookbook

*121 Foolproof, Delicious and Easy-to-Follow Recipes | The Smart Diet to Weight Loss Without Food Restrictions*

## Kelly Jason

# Disclaimer

© Copyright 2020 by Kelly Jason - All rights reserved.

The following eBook is reproduced below with the goal of providing information that is as accurate and reliable as possible. Regardless, purchasing this eBook can be seen as consent to the fact that both the publisher and the author of this book are in no way experts on the topics discussed within and that any recommendations or suggestions that are made herein are for entertainment purposes only. Professionals should be consulted as needed prior to undertaking any of the action endorsed herein.

This declaration is deemed fair and valid by both the American Bar Association and the Committee of Publishers Association and is legally binding throughout the United States.

Furthermore, the transmission, duplication, or reproduction of any of the following work including specific information will be considered an illegal act irrespective of if it is done electronically or in print. This extends to creating a secondary or tertiary copy of the work or a recorded copy and is only allowed with the express written consent from the Publisher. All additional right reserved.

The information in the following pages is broadly considered a truthful and accurate account of facts and as such, any inattention, use, or misuse of the information in question by the reader will render any resulting actions solely under their purview. There are no scenarios in which the publisher or the original author of this work can be in any fashion deemed liable for any hardship or damages that may befall them after undertaking information described herein.

Additionally, the information in the following pages is intended only for informational purposes and should thus be thought of as universal. As befitting its nature, it is presented without assurance regarding its prolonged validity or interim quality. Trademarks that are mentioned are done without written consent and can in no way be considered an endorsement from the trademark holder.

# Table Of Contents

**Table Of Contents** — 4

**INTRODUCTION** — 1

**Watch Your Weight Go Down with Weight Watchers** — 3

    How do weight observers work? — 4

    What's the default behind the dumbbells? — 4

    Society — 5

    Evolution — 5

    Their commitment to fitness — 6

**Benefits Of Weight Watchers Lifestyle** — 8

    The nutritional benefits of quinoa for weight monitoring — 8

    Benefits of weight watchers' privileges — 9

| | |
|---|---:|
| Benefits of the Weight Watchers program | 10 |
| Lifestyle conscious of weight-conscious | 12 |

## The FIRST World Diet To Have Weekly Group Support Also Online    13

| | |
|---|---:|
| Why Weight Watchers Work | 13 |
| How Weight Watchers Can Help You | 16 |
| Meetings | 18 |

## All Food Groups Included, No Food Restrictions For Weight Loss Without Suffering    20

| | |
|---|---:|
| Healthy weight management means balancing food groups | 22 |
| Calorie restriction for weight loss explained | 24 |
| Maintaining a healthy caloric level | 24 |
| Calculate the amount of calorie restriction | 25 |
| Reduces calories | 25 |

## Weight Watchers Points System — 27

    What are they? — 27

    A healthy way to get a diet — 28

    Weight Watchers Evaluation List — 31

## WW And Mind: HOW This Lifestyle Will Definitely Change Your Mindset — 33

    Meditation for weight loss and more natural control — 33

    Proper Mindset — 35

## 121 Yummy Recipes (Breakfast, Lunch And Dinner) For YOU And YOUR Family — 37

    Breakfast — 38

    Lunch — 57

    Dinner — 76

| | |
|---|---|
| Sides | 93 |
| Salads | 108 |
| Fish and Seafood | 121 |
| Poultry and Beef | 134 |
| Appetizers and Snacks | 149 |
| Desserts | 160 |
| Sauces and Seasonings | 174 |

**28 Different Introductory WW Day Plans For Beginners** — 179

| | |
|---|---|
| Shopping Guide and Food List | 190 |

**Weight Watchers Top 15 Tips And Tricks** — 198

**Conclusion** — 203

# INTRODUCTION

Thank you for downloading this fantastic guide, "Weight Watchers Freestyle Cookbook."

If you're looking for both weight and nutrition, this weight Watcher easy cookbook can be a great tool.

The recipes you'll see in the Weight Watcher's freestyle Cookbook include a full range of sauces, pieces of bread, soups, meat, poultry, fish and vegetables, portions of pasta, vegetables, cereals and potato preparations, and most important. It includes desserts, meals, and recipes in the book refer to healthy and healthy eating, but many of your favorite foods may not be part of your diet.

Customers around the world have admired many internationally inspired recipes. So Weight Watcher Freestyle Cook is quality and quantity in terms of recipes, but the nutritional focus sets it apart from the regular cookbook.

Breakdown of independent books is a heavyweight observation, which includes calories, fat, saturated fat, cholesterol, sodium, carbohydrates, fiber, protein, and calcium.

The Freestyle Watchers Cookbook is very balanced with recipes for many diets. Whether you are a busy single expert, who only has time for a quick meal after work, or a housekeeper who wants a for the family of four, this book has everything.

# WEIGHT WATCHERS FREESTYLE COOKBOOK

Besides the highest quality of the Cook Watcher Freestyle, there are a few small features very useful:

- 121 Interesting recipes (breakfast, lunch, and dinner) for you and your family
- 28 WW introductory programs WW beginner's introduction
- Losing Weight While Having Fun with Weight Watchers Tips (Smart Score Program)

Therefore, if you are after a free cookbook and weight tracker, it is undoubtedly a choice that will bring you the same variety and tastes of any cookbook available on the market, while looking for your weight and health.

Weight Watchers is more than just a weight loss program. Observers allow you to travel in groups, with people trying to lose weight. Most important, diet plans are sustainable. Unlike many raw diets outside the world, foods that provide temporary results and can have potentially dangerous side effects are a safe alternative for viewers.

## Let's begin!

# Watch Your Weight Go Down with Weight Watchers

Weight Watchers is a diet program that inspires and guides people towards healthier choices so they can live life to the fullest. Supported by Oprah Winfrey's appreciation and more, it has a system that divides complex nutrition information into simple numbers called points.

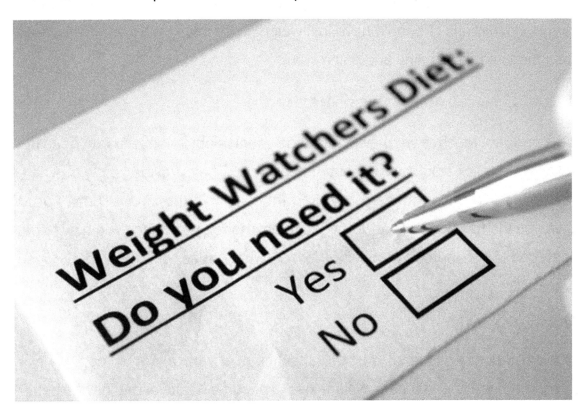

The Weight Watchers menu has all the foods on its list, but with these points, it is assigned to each meal. The goal is to gradually move towards a healthier diet, consisting of lower protein, fruits, and vegetables, but lower levels of sugar and fat. Weight Watchers is one of the best weight loss programs available. Given the ease of doing this, that you can eat real food and the support provided, you can easily understand why.

## How do weight observers work?

Weight Watchers has a good track record and has been in the weightlifting business for over 40 years. This long history gives credibility to weight loss programs. Millions of people have lost weight in the plan, and it works because it supports eating healthy and doing work.

## What's the default behind the dumbbells?

This program teaches you how to manage your weight in the long run, does not give you a quick solution you cannot cope with. They provide you with all the information you need to learn how to eat healthily in the long run, they don't give you the functional foods you need to eat, nor do they teach you how to eat real food. This approach to weight loss is what causes many people to lose weight.

Discover more

The diet industry has received more attention over time, and most people have recognized the importance of weight loss to become healthier and have a better personality. However, very few organizations in the industry have been genuinely successful. One is the dumbbell, which has been around for a long time and has grown steadily to this day. What matters to the success of the Watcher's success?

## Society

Unbelievable, but the sense of community among those trying to lose weight is one of the most important things behind the great success of observers. Sharing your personal experience of success and failure with others gives you a thrilling and humbling feeling.

Most of the time, people trying to lose weight do not receive support because there is no home assistance system. When you are in the weightlifting program, the obligation is made during the meeting with other team members, and like a special connection between people are different in everything except one thing in common - their desire for health. Each weightlifting program has its own set of obstacles and must support each other to stay motivated and encouraged to continue their program.

## Evolution

Weight watchers are following a successful model and achieving weight loss goals. However, this model does not go beyond development. While participation in meetings is crucial for participants, this weight loss program offers the perfect options for regular meetings for people with a hectic schedule and for those who do not feel comfortable at meetings. This is where online forums, support groups, and message forums come into play. However, the evolution of the program is not limited to online forums, support groups, and message boards. The dumbbells also incorporated an evaluation system that allows members to evaluate and evaluate their performance according to food requirements and standards, regardless of the need to weigh their food or the number of calories they consume. How is it? We all live in a crowded, fast-paced world, where there are a lot of problems and professionals so diet professionals can closely monitor calorie consumption.

The Watchers website is an excellent example of how the program will meet the diverse needs of people. If you have not visited the Weight Watchers website, try to check it out and use the fantastic information and valuable information you offer.

## Their commitment to fitness

The weight loss program also believes that weight loss goals are not just achieved through diet. The deeper the result, the faster you get when you combine diet and exercise. That this weight loss program believes in the importance of physical fitness and exercise, along with proper nutrition and proper mentality when talking about diet, is another reason for their great success.

Weight Watchers is one of the many diets and weight loss programs we have on the market today. They have created a reputation that is, above all else, is something that must be taken seriously. Every month we see new programs coming out, but Weight Watchers never fails to deliver consistent and visible results to the people watching it. No other weight loss program has claimed this for as long as Weight Watchers has.

When you combine the above three with pre-packaged Weight Watchers, extended, and healthy recipes, you will find lasting success.

# Benefits Of Weight Watchers Lifestyle

## The nutritional benefits of quinoa for weight monitoring

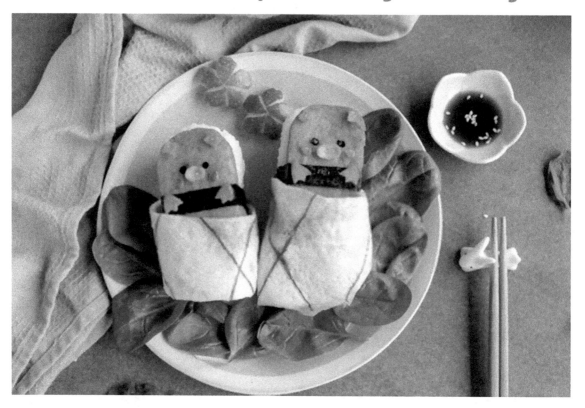

Weight loss is quite substantial, and what I hate most is how you will have to change your eating and eating habits. I think most experts would agree with me if I said that you don't have to kill yourself to shed extra pounds. There is certainly a way to get the weight you always wanted; without the quality of the food you give.

Quinoa is famous not only among health enthusiasts but also among weight watchers. There are many nutritional benefits of quinoa that you can read online, and let's quickly summarize them all. Grains such as grains contain twice as much protein as regular cereals but have fewer carbohydrates, healthier fats, fiber, phosphorus, calcium, and iron. Now, this is an excellent news. This is a necessity for overseas dumbbells. However, it is unfortunate that the benefits of quinoa are not recognized by the general population. This is the most nutritious seed you can ever have.

Manganese and copper are also the nutritional benefits of the quinoa you can get. These two minerals work together as antioxidants to get rid of the body of free radicals. Free radicals are believed to cause cancer and other diseases. It also accelerates the aging process.

What are the other nutritional benefits of quinoa for weight watchers? Besides the fact that quinoa is full of nutrients, vitamins, and minerals, one thing I like is that it helps you feel full. What do you say Quinoa carbohydrates are slowly released into the body, which means that after eating a specific type of food, you will not get an energy rush? Don't worry about your sweet cravings, because if you include quinoa in your diet, it will disappear. Eating quinoa helps you control hunger.

## Benefits of weight watchers' privileges

The weight loss program has been around for a long time, and there have been thousands of success stories of some people who were in a weight loss regime and have lost weight and kept it off. This weight loss program may be the most popular and well-known diet available today and have a unique history for most other programs. We want to take a look at how Weight Watchers Point can benefit you. When Weight Watchers first started operating, they did not have a rating system, and there were several diet books. But they have updated their diet and now have a very easy to use a point system.

Whatever you eat and consume depends on the number of points you get, and depending on weight, age, and other factors, you are allowed a certain amount of points per day. This makes it less cumbersome when you add points and knows precisely what to keep.

Another benefit of using the points system is that you will find out which foods are best to eat and, as a rule, things that grow are much better than processed foods. Weight Watchers Scorecard also gives you a certain amount of oil and water that you need to consume daily, as it helps boost your metabolism and also helps you lose weight faster.

Keep in mind that if you are looking for an easy-to-follow diet plan, you should consider the Observers Weight Score Plan.

## Benefits of the Weight Watchers program

Today, many of us have probably heard about dumbbells. Weight Watchers is one of the most effective and popular weight loss programs for those who have to lose weight and have benefited from thousands from this program. However, this program will not be suitable for everyone, despite its many benefits. Therefore, these programs have limitations and disadvantages. Before deciding on a decision to use it, consider all the advantages and disadvantages of this weight Watcher program.

The advantages of this scheme are the following:

1. There are no restrictions on the type of food to be consumed, so there is no prohibited food. This app allows you to eat whatever you want but in moderation. The advantage is that you can still enjoy all your favorite foods in smaller portions than before. There are no banned foods in the Weight Watcher app, so you don't have to eat your favorite food.

2. Your group is led by a leader who is aware of the specific nutritional needs of each member so that you have a good knowledge of diet, eating well, and consuming each one day.

3. Meetings are flexible. So, you can probably bring your kids in front of your sessions. You don't have to worry about leaving them home alone because you want to improve on weight issues.

4- The Watchers Weight program supports the achievable results. Therefore, you may notice a slow and continuous weight loss in the body. Expect to lose at least one kg after one week of enrollment and grow more each week. The more effort and discipline you have, the more weight you can lose.

5. Training is given on how to control your food portions. With the Watcher Weight program, you learn how to measure and track your diet so that even if you stop attending meetings, knowledge will remain with you throughout your life so you can keep up with what you eat daily. Control your weight.

## Lifestyle conscious of weight-conscious

The key to success in weight loss and weight control is understanding change is a permanent change in lifestyle and not a unique event. Controlling your weight or maintaining your weight from now on is a continuous process that you must take full responsibility for. Having a successful lifestyle leads to more pressure than anything else than dieting and what is your goal in achieving your weight. It's about reaching your goal of losing weight and having a plan to get there.

Living a healthier and healthier lifestyle than what you eat is what you are. It's about empowering you to take control of your life and create your future. The benefits are enormous. You look and feel better, you become healthier, you increase self-esteem, you increase self-esteem, and you can achieve the other goal you want in life.

For the weight observer, having a weight loss program that includes a balanced diet and proper exercise program, along with daily meditation exercises, is the best way to build your mind, body, and emotion to make you healthier and thinner.

# The FIRST World Diet To Have Weekly Group Support Also Online

## Why Weight Watchers Work

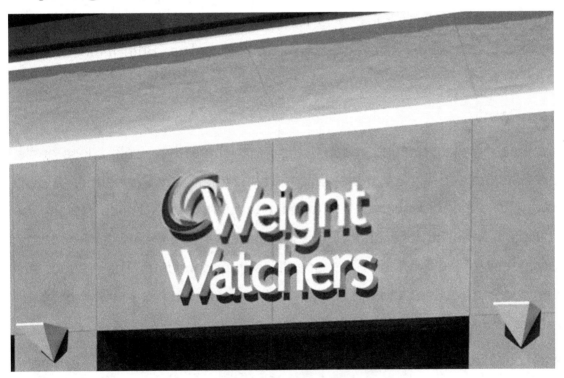

Weight Watchers is a program that helps participants lose weight. This app is different because it allows participants to buy and cook their food options. It has proven to be active and is a good diet option for those who want to lose weight and those who can only gain a few extra pounds to get rid of it. The dumbbells also have a separate program for people with specific nutritional needs.

## Online Or Face To Face

There are two ways to register for Weight Watchers. The first and most traditional way is to find and attend meetings. Meetings are generally held once a week and include discussions, updates, resource sharing, and weekly weights. Online weight tracking is for those who are upset at face-to-face meetings or prefer the convenience of working online. Both methods have proven to work.

## Food Points

To create a weight-bearing work, participants share their weight loss goals, eating habits, and activity preferences. Then, the system generates a daily average score. This average is found considering how much weight the participants want to lose and what their current body weight is. Each day, participants record the foods and quantities they consume. These foods are given constant values, and the objective of the participant is to stay within the average range allowed for that day.

Teach participants to eat healthily and understand what to avoid. For example, a piece of cheese can have 12 points. If a participant has only 20 points a day, the cheese will earn more than half of its daily value. They can still eat hamburgers if they want, but they only have 8 points to use for the rest of the meals and snacks before they sign up for the diet. But instead, if that person had a cup of boiled chicken rice and spinach, he could only use 7 or 8 points, which could mean more options for other meals. It teaches participants which foods are worse or better than others.

Those who sign up for Weight Watchers are also offered a certain number of pre-set points that they can use at any time. These points can be added to the daily total or saved by the end of each week.

## Activity Score

Activity points are used to reward rewards. Many different forms of exercise, from running, swimming, to gardening, are considered acceptable. The duration and intensity of these activities determine how many events are assigned. These points can be used to remove excess nutrient points. The more active the participants, the more flexible the food choices. Encourage participants to have good eating habits with good sports habits.

## Weigh-Ins

Weight Watchers Weight Watchers happen once a week. For face-to-face meetings, participants weigh their members as a form of transplant. Weights are recorded, and we recommend weight loss or weight gain for the week, if necessary. To sing online, participants enter their weight weekly on the computer.

## Resources

Weight Watchers provides many resources for its members. From recipes to tips and advice, members can have information on how to feed and stay healthy at the same time. Weight watchers do not do much about eating and the best ways to lose weight and create wholesome routines for many people in a variety of living conditions.

## Maintenance

Another unique aspect of the Weight Watchers program is that it teaches participants to maintain their weight and how to continue with their new healthy lifestyle while doing it while training.

Members do what is best for them. Incense and why this app becomes second nature and instead teaches members-only pre-made foods to choose the best segments and options.

## How Weight Watchers Can Help You

## Track Weight

Weight Watchers is the largest and also the world's leading weight loss company. Founded in 1963, the successful company focuses its diet plans on three simple concepts.

First, a successful diet plan should limit the number of calories you consume; secondly, exercise is an essential component of any diet plan and, thirdly, supporting a team that helps you make good choices and guide you towards your ultimate goal. To guide... The company has more than 1.5 million members in Diet Watchers Weight and more than 50,000 sessions worldwide each week.

## How it works

The weight Watchers system operates by "points." Scores are based on the calories of a product that makes this design look weird. Although this is a relatively simple concept, calorie reduction is the main ingredient in weight loss. The dumbbells currently have two alternative diets, Flex Plan and Core Plan.

As you expect, Flex Plan offers you more nutritional alternatives. This diet follows the points system and, because each food is assigned a "point" value, you can eat all your favorite foods, control the amount of food. The tips that are offered to you on a given day will be determined by sex, age, weight, and height. It is a natural diet that you only follow with the little mathematics needed to add and manage your daily scores.

The main diet goes beyond the system of necessary privileges. It is suitable for people who do not want to calculate everything because it is based on the consumption of healthy foods. You can choose from all the essential food groups, including fruits, vegetables, cereals, starches, lean meats, poultry, and dairy products, and you can eat all "acceptable" foods and even once. Live with a snack (provided it is in a controlled quantity).

Viewers encourage regular exercise, and their website, available at http://www.weightwatchers.com, has several different options. One of the changes to their plan is that, instead of punishing the diet for not exercising, the program encourages athletes by adding extra points.

## Meetings

Another key to the Weight Watchers program is participation in conferences. While you can use the online application, assistance, and guidance from in-person meetings can significantly increase your success rate. It is always helpful to always hear the actual experiences of other diets and find out about their struggles with weight and make the lifestyle changes needed to maintain your weight.

Diets for weight watchers do not work for everyone. The core is a calorie-based diet. There may be potential health problems related to weight problems, such as adrenal fatigue, carbohydrate sensitivity, low serotonin levels, or intestinal parasites. Also, since the members need to stay at one point as a whole, they must eat an adequate diet so that they can consume all the nutrients and vitamins needed for health.

Sometimes counting points can be tiring or can lead to food remedies. The cost of participating in all weightlifting programs can be very costly. The registration fee is $ 30 for the online application and $ 17 per month, which in addition to your food, depending on the area you live in, usually costs $ 10 per week.

The big question is whether people can lose weight with the Watchers Weight programs. In a 2003 study published in the Journal of the American Medical Association (JAMA) (and funded by Watchers), people who followed the Weight Watchers assessment program lost an average of six kilos after two years. Diets that participate in at least 78% of weekly sessions have nearly doubled their weight loss to 11 kilograms, so you have to take seriously all aspects of the plan to be successful.

# All Food Groups Included, No Food Restrictions For Weight Loss Without Suffering

When you want to change your diet to lose weight or to improve your health, you need to make sure that all 4 groups of foods are balanced. If you can create the necessary dietary measures to include all of these nutritional groups, the effects on your health and weight will be very positive.

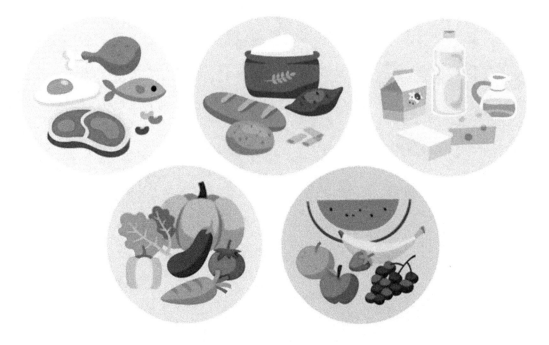

1. Proteins provide the body with what it needs for healthy growth. Proteins also govern metabolism and hormonal functions. Metabolism is an essential factor in controlling your weight. The more metabolism you have, the more calories you burn each day. Therefore, if you get enough protein, you may have healthier metabolism and burn more calories each day, you will need less diet to lose weight.

You can find protein in foods such as chicken, eggs, fish, and dairy. The disadvantage of these foods is that they tend to have a higher fat content, so you can avoid foods high in protein, such as cereals and vegetables that provide protein. Overeating protein can have negative consequences, especially kidney stones and gout. The key is to consume them in balance with other foods.

2. Fats and oils are usually bad for you. However, these are an essential part of your diet. They are called essential fatty acids and are found in fish, nuts, and seeds. They are necessary because the body cannot produce them alone and are a vital ingredient for our overall biological system.

3. Fruits and vegetables provide vitamins and minerals, fiber, and many other active substances. Most people believe that only fresh organic vegetables are worth consuming, but frozen vegetables and roots also provide valuable nutrients. Consuming fruits and vegetables every day can boost the body's immune system, improve the appearance of your skin, plus all aspects of your health.

4. Carbohydrates are found in both processed and complex forms. Processed carbohydrates should be largely avoided and include foods such as white pasta, cakes, and bread. They have a lot of sugar and saturated fat. Complex carbohydrates are found in foods such as vegetables, wheat, and couscous. They are crucial to providing the energy needed for the body to function. Without carbs, you will probably feel tired and lethargic.

5. Fiber is the fifth food group that should be included in your balanced diet. Its primary purpose is to clean your bowels and keep you organized. Without enough fiber, your body will work to clean up toxins and waste. It is also very effective in preventing multiple diseases.

By eating the right balance of these five food groups every day, you pay to keep your whole body healthy.

## Healthy weight management means balancing food groups

Many diet programs focus on eliminating specific food groups. Reducing each group of dietary needs presents certain risks over time.

High protein diets are because they are famous for a long time to reduce your hunger problems. It allows you to eat less over a certain period and, in turn, consume fewer calories.

Carbohydrates are known as fatty foods. The calories in all meals are to blame. Carbohydrates are the source of energy for the body and muscles. If we eliminate all carbs, we increase the risk of losing power to an excessively inactive level.

Lack of physical activity and exercise determines fat storage and does not reduce weight for our efforts. On the contrary, this is a good line trying to determine the level of carbohydrates we need. Crossing the line and consuming carbohydrates is very easy. The result is not weight loss again.

High protein diets usually include animal protein and fat. These indicate the risk of increased cholesterol levels.

It is essential that active people want to manage their weight, including breakfast and lunch, which are either full carbohydrates for energy and protein for fullness or full sensation, as well as nutritional ingredients such as whole grains, milk, turkey on bread and pasta with meat sauce.

To meet the energy needs of an active adult, you should eat high-protein foods, such as peanut butter, bean salad, or tofu, with pasta at each meal.

Beans, soybeans, or other plant proteins are essential to provide adequate amounts of protein to perform muscle maintenance, iron supply and prevent anemia, containing the amount of zinc needed to stimulate recovery and immunity. Replacing natural foods with protein supplements limits the number of nutrients and nutrients needed in whole foods.

To encourage healthy muscles, you need adequate protein, extra carbohydrates, and resistance training, such as dumbbells. Carbohydrates nourish your muscles and provide you with the energy required to stimulate the level of energy needed for a healthy workout and healthy lifestyle.

It is generally accepted that a healthy adult needs 9.9 grams of protein per kilogram of healthy weight. For example, if you weigh 160 pounds and want to get the highest protein, you need 144 grams of protein. This can be expressed in a one-day diet that includes a quarter of low-fat milk. One tin and eight ounces of chicken breast.

## Calorie restriction for weight loss explained

Poor diets, low carbohydrate diets, and low-fat diets can cause rapid weight loss with supplements, dietary supplements, and other products. Still, the real secret is to lose weight permanently, limiting your total daily calorie intake. It is nutritious while still providing food.

## Maintaining a healthy caloric level

Keep in mind that too few calories in the body can lead to health problems. Calories are the energy from foods that the body needs for normal functions. Calorie energy is the fuel that fuels every action the body performs from lifting a finger to participating in a trilateral.

The primary sources of calories are nutrients, i.e., carbohydrates, proteins, and fats, although the amount of calories and, therefore, the energy provided by each food source varies. These calories are converted into physical energy or fat stored in the body, which will remain as fat unless you attract it as energy storage. Therefore, to lose weight, it is necessary to reduce total calories daily, increase physical activity, or, preferably, both, which in turn lead to faster burning of calories.

## Calculate the amount of calorie restriction

Despite the very complex calorie calculations used by many weight loss professionals, the idea is relatively simple. If you eat more calories than calories burned for energy, you gain weight faster. Even the basic formula is natural to know exactly how many calories to lose weight to consume and burn.

Keep in mind that one cup of body fat is 3,500 calories. So, if you want to lose 1 kilogram, you have to burn 3,500 calories. Now suppose you want to lose 1kg every week.

Just divide the number of calories in kilograms by the number of days (7 / 7,500) to reach 500, which indicates the name of calories you need to reduce from your daily diet.

## Reduces calories

Contrary to popular belief, cutting calories from a daily diet is not a disappointing exercise. The secret of success in limiting calories is the gradual decrease in dietary changes required instead of a full 180-degree turn. You will end up with the pressures of starvation to such an extent that food will inevitably turn into a square.

Experts recommend three steps to limit efficient calories:

- Avoid heat burns during the day, such as after-dinner ice cream bowls, lunch breaks at a snack bar, and leave with extra cream in the morning.

- Replace calorie-rich foods with a low-calorie option. Choose an option that will continue to appeal to you, so you don't miss out. For example, choose a soft drink instead of iced caramel coffee.

- Reduce the size because it is clear that smaller sizes lead to fewer calories. Instead of 1 glass of pasta, choose only half a cup.

Stringent calorie restriction must be combined with moderate exercise and healthy lifestyle habits to keep weight loss results. Remember that this trinity of weight loss is practical because one of the missing elements is destroying your efforts to look back and feel healthy again.

# Weight Watchers Points System

## What are they?

|  | Green | Blue | Purple |
|---|---|---|---|
| The Lowdown | Less zero point foods, higher daily points budget to use on other foods | Freestyle plan. Medium amount of zero point foods, medium daily points budget | More zero point foods, less daily points to spend on other foods |
| Minimum Daily Points Budget | 30 | 23 | 16 |
| Number of Zero Point Foods | 100+ | 200+ | 300+ |
| Zero Point Food Categories | Fruits, Non-starchy Vegetables | Fruits, Most Vegetables (adds corn and peas, but not potatoes, avocados), Eggs, Skinless Chicken and Turkey Breast, Fish/Shellfish, Nonfat Plain Yogurt/Soy Yogurt, Beans and Legumes, Tofu and | Fruits, Vegetables (but not avocados), Eggs, Skinless Chicken and Turkey Breast, Fish/Shellfish, Nonfat Plain Yogurt/Soy Yogurt, Beans and Legumes, Tofu and Tempeh, Potatoes and Sweet Potatoes, Whole Wheat Pasta/certain Veggie Pastas, Brown Rice and Wild Rice, Oats, Other whole |

The weightlifting program is a successful weight loss program, with a focus on balanced nutrition, low-fat content, and good exercise. This is a diet plan in which each food item has a certain amount of energy called "weight loss points," for example 100 grams of white bread containing about six of them, while the same slice the cake has 10 points of the same weight.

Some computers can calculate your nutritional value and your meals alone. It is based on a system that practically calculates the number of calories, the amount of hot fiber, and the amount of burning fat.

And so to create a unique, but very profound and creative way of saying the value of the food energy we consume. The study found that people who use this method and follow a diet lose, on average, about 6 kilos in two years.

But remember it's an average, most engaged and even lost 50 pounds. He also advises overweight or people with a family history of problems that can be caused by overweight, such as diabetes or heart disease, which can significantly affect their health.

The highlight of this program is that you don't have to kill any of your favorite foods. Another advantage of the application itself is that it is very flexible and can be adapted to your lifestyle.

In short, this is a program that allows you to lose weight even without sacrificing any of your favorite foods.

## A healthy way to get a diet

Observers are one of the most popular weight loss programs on the market today. People who were part of the program know that it works. With millions of members around the world, this is not popular, but it has helped countless men and women control their weight. Whether it is 10 kilograms or 100 kilograms, the members managed to lose weight in a very healthy way using the weight system for weight observers.

According to the weight loss plan, a portion is granted based on the portion size, the number of calories, the fiber content, and the amount of fat in the food. Foods with a higher level of fat mean more fiber points. The daily score of each person is determined by the goal of weight loss and body weight. The weight scoring system is a very creative and easy way to lose weight healthily.

Wondering if Weight Watchers will work? Here are three main reasons that led to the successful reduction of weight loss program members:

### It's easy

While this sounds simple, it is true. To succeed in this program, you do not need to be a diet and exercise expert. Learn how to read food labels while you're at the grocery store, and you're on the road. The program uses a rating system, which determines the number of carbohydrates, calories, fats, etc., for each food item you want to eat. Be below the limit

### Eat the foods you like

For those who love a specific type of food, Weight Watchers works because it does not eliminate a particular type of food. For example, like Atkins, which eliminates carbohydrates, this program teaches you to eat in moderation. If you can't give up something like chocolate or bread, you don't have to sacrifice yourself. You have to eat within range and eat them in moderation, rather than getting rid of them. This makes success much more comfortable.

### You will see real results

Losing 2 kilograms a week helps people plan to lose weight. When people are encouraged by their progress, they are more likely to stick to the program.

**Can you eat whatever you want?**

One of the promotional benefits of following the Observer rating system is that it allows you to eat whatever you want - as long as the food is allocated to your daily places. To some, this may seem unbelievable. How can you eat whatever you want and lose weight further? The truth is a little more complicated.

**How do weight observer assessments work?**

In essence, the WW rating system is a way to count calories. Each "point" has about 50 calories, although there are some variations. For example, a diet high in fiber can have 100 calories, but it only has 1 point.

When you start the weight Watchers program, you are awarded points, and you must limit your daily use to this number. You can score points for sports, as well as 35 flexible points that you can use throughout the week - either as an extra 5 points per day or as a great meal. Some people decide not to use those areas at all.

As the day goes on, you will calculate the amount of food you eat and add them throughout the day, making sure you are no more than your share.

**Can you eat whatever you want using the Weight Watchers score?**

The short answer is yes. Of course, you can only do this if you have enough food for your day. For example, you cannot eat an additional amount of McDonald's, a small pizza, and 12 candy a day. Theoretically, you can eat nothing but sweet and yet lose weight. You will be limited to the number of candies that match the score range. Of course, you will probably be hungry during the day, because the candy will not hold you ultimately.

## Weight Watchers Evaluation List

Weight watchers have been around for many years, and the list of spots for Weight Watchers is becoming more and more popular with people on a diet. It is one of the most popular weight loss programs overseas and not only offers weight loss products and supplements for weight loss but also has a unique dating and support system that provides more diet programs.

The best thing about the dumbbell list is that it can be used by anyone, regardless of whether it is in the dumbbell program or not. However, finding food tips can be a daunting task. The complex calculation of calories, fat, and fiber content takes advantage of that particular food.

If you go through the list of weight lifting tips, however, food is already shared with you. All you have to do is add what you want to eat, score a little if needed so that you can earn points daily, and that's it!

The number of points you can get per day varies depending on your weight. For example, if you weigh between 175 and 199 pounds, you can gain 22 to 27 points per day. If you weigh more or less, you may have more or fewer points. This works because as soon as you lose weight, you will fall into a lower weight category - and thus, you will earn fewer points. The less you eat, the fewer calories you will get, and the more weight you will lose. This is an easy way to shed pounds!

The list of weight evaluators is the best way to track. Let's look at a typical light meal and count the benefits. For dinner, let's say you have a passion for seafood.

- 1 6 salmon fillets = 7 points
- 12 spears of asparagus = 0 points
- 1 roll of each type = 3 points
- 1 tall glass of sweet tea = 2 points
- 1 tablespoon of frozen ice cream for dessert = 2 points

Notice how generous I was with this sweet tooth at dinner. You have salmon, asparagus, and a roll. Sweet tea can always be replaced with zero water, and ice cream is an ice cream that you would have avoided if you wanted to. Even with the good things added, you only use 14 points for dinner. This gives you some other tips to use for the rest of your days!

As you can see, the Weight Watchers checklist is fascinating for excellent reasons. It allows you to eat what you want until you overeat. If you count all your points, your weight loss program will be a surprise, and your kilos will melt!

# WW And Mind: HOW This Lifestyle Will Definitely Change Your Mindset

Meditation for weight loss and more natural control

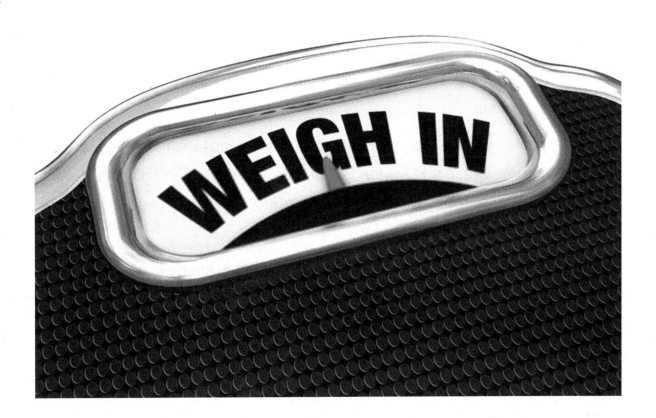

You may not realize how vital personal goals are, especially in terms of self-improvement and personal development. Weight loss and weight control are in both groups and are certainly a kind of self-help.

As with any set goal, the belief that you can and will achieve it gives you over ninety percent of the path to achievement. What you think and believe about reaching a specific goal is far more important than the action needed to achieve it. As the renowned author, **Napoleon Hill**, said: *"Any mind can imagine and believe it can achieve."*

When it comes to your mind to think and act in a positive way to reach the goal, most people turn to statements and statements. But there is a problem with these techniques.

Most people who use them get inferior results because statements are used while they are awake and aware. In this case, the usual distractions are much more than the mind's ability to work in a specific and challenging way, which in turn hinders the desired results.

On the other hand, when meditation is used alongside affirmations, affirmations become hundreds of times more effective because they work at the subconscious level of the mind. At the conscious level of consciousness, the brain can clearly focus on the desired goal and can lead you to achieve it much faster, no matter what the goal is.

Positive affirmations, such as "I enjoy constant weight gain in my normal bodyweight of XXX pounds," have a more profound impact on my mind when I rest in a quiet state of mind, where the subconscious mind can understand and can guide you. Your weight control program will. Take appropriate action, especially when you can imagine how you will look and feel about this weight.

From this moment on, your subconscious plays a vital role in keeping you from reaching your weight loss goal and keeping your weight there once. By default, you will unconsciously notice that you eat less, eat better for yourself, want to make more effort, and generally better health.

Dedicating less than 15 minutes a day to a simple meditation exercise will not only benefit you from the weight loss program, but it can also lead you to a healthier, happier, more productive life without stress.

## Proper Mindset

Follow a nutritionally, scientifically proven, lean diet. Get into physical activity or participate in an exercise approved by specialists. Use a system to measure your progress. These are just some of the most common tips you will get from experts when looking for weight loss and maintaining your ideal body.

And for fast weight loss results, they recommend the use of a comprehensive fitness program that includes virtually all of these techniques that complement all other fitness components and that all work well in helping you work toward your fitness goals... It is expected that you can achieve the desired results, as long as you follow the steps as faithfully as possible.

If this is easy and simple, then why do people still fail? Even those who are trying to be careful with a fitness program for weight training find it difficult. Some who were very eager to get started refused to work. Others even cheat or refuse instructions. However, others offer diet plans and exercises that reduce fat intake.

So, have you tried many different fitness programs, but have not yet achieved the desired results? An essential step that can be missed is getting the right thinking. To help you reach your weight loss goals, experts have realized that the mind must first function in the body.

This requires a lot of motivation and inspiration to overcome all the fitness challenges. Eliminating the board of directors cannot be achieved simply by administering a reduced food intake, by capturing loyalty and by providing calories per meal or after each routine and even overcoming the limitations of the body so that you can adjust it. Rotate or repeat workouts. How your mind works is also essential for all these improvements.

Make sure your mind is paying attention to it. Get motivated and get inspired by learning how to get rid of blockchain. Argue and support "no" in any way you do or in any container you say, developing a realistic but enthusiastic perspective. You have the right thinking, and you can overcome all the challenges and be encouraged to continue on the road, not only to reach your ideal weight but also to live a healthier and more active life.

# 121 Yummy Recipes (Breakfast, Lunch And Dinner) For YOU And YOUR Family

Whether you are cooking for two or ten, or even more, you want your weight watchers' meals recipes to be absolutely delicious. You also want them to be fast, easy and above all quick healthy meal ideas. You do not want to rely on eating out frequently, nor do you want to be stuck preparing boxed, bagged, or frozen meals all of the time.

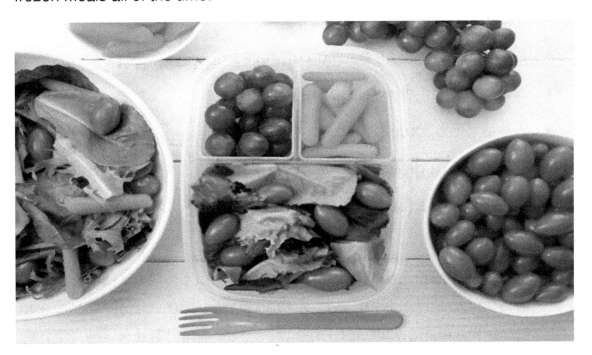

In this chapter, I have shared over hundred recipes you can try out. They are quick and fast to prepare with an average time of 6 minutes.

## Breakfast

# Beef and Bacon "Rice" with Pine Nuts

### Ingredients

- ½ head cauliflower
- 8 scallions, thinly sliced
- 2/3 cup (100 g) diced green pepper
- 1 tablespoon (28 g) butter
- 1 tablespoon (15 ml) olive oil
- 1 teaspoon chicken bouillon granules
- ¼ cup (60 ml) dry white wine
- ¼ cup (30 g) crumbled blue cheese
- ¼ cup (25 g) grated Parmesan cheese
- 2 tablespoons (30 ml) heavy cream

### Instructions

- Put cauliflower using a food processor with a razor blade. Put it in a microwave oven, add a tablespoon (30 ml) of water, and cover the microwave for 7 minutes over high heat.

- While cooking, chop the onion and sauté the pepper. In a large, heavy fish, over medium heat, begin to marinate onions and peppers in butter and oil.

- When the oven is "submerged", remove the cauliflower and drain it. When the green pepper begins to soften, dart the cauliflower at the fish and mix. Then mix in Bowl, white wine, blue cheese, parmesan and heavy cream. Cook and serve for another 3-4 minutes.

**Yield:**

5 servings

Each with 4 grams of carbohydrates and 1 gram of fiber, for a total of 3 grams of usable carbohydrates and 4 grams of protein

## Apple Pie Breakfast Farro

**Ingredients**

- 8.8 ounces (249 g) quick-cooking dry farro
- 3 McIntosh apples, or any favorite apple, cored and chopped
- ¼ cup (48 g) Sucanat or
- 1½ teaspoons ground cinnamon, plus optional extra for garnish
- 1 teaspoon pure vanilla extract
- 1 cup (235 ml) plain or vanilla vegan milk, warmed, as needed

- 1 or 2 recipes of nuts from Seed and Nut Ice Cream
- Pure maple syrup, optional

**Instructions**

- Boil a large pot of water. Add the farro and boil again. Lower the heat to medium low and expose. Cook for 10 to 12 minutes until al dente or consistency is reached. Drain and reserve.

- Place the chopped apples, lettuce or brown sugar and cinnamon in the same large pot used to cook the farro. Heat to medium-high, stirring to combine. Once the apples release their moisture, reduce the heat to medium and cook until the apples are tender, about 10 to 15 minutes, stirring constantly. Keep in mind that the cooking time will vary depending on the part of apple and the type of apple you use. You're looking for tender bits, but not applesauce.

- Drop the pot and mix the vanilla into the apples. Add the cooked grain into the apples and serve immediately, topping each serving with as much of the warm milk as desired. Top each serving with a handful of nuts, extra cinnamon, and maple syrup if desired.

**Yield:**

4 to 6 servings

**Protein content per serving:**

19 g

# Chicken-Almond "Rice"

**Ingredients**

- ½ head cauliflower
- ½ medium onion, chopped
- 2 tablespoons (28 g) butter, divided
- 1 tablespoon (6 g) chicken bouillon granules
- 1 teaspoon poultry seasoning
- ¼ cup (60 ml) dry white wine
- ¼ cup (30 g) sliced or slivered almonds

**Instructions**

- Run the cauliflower using a food processor with a razor blade. Put the cauliflower in a microwave oven, a few tablespoons (30 ml) of water, cover and
- Microwave for 7 minutes.
- While cooking, heat the onion in a large butter (14 g) in a large skillet over medium heat.

- When the cauliflower is over, remove it from the microwave, drain it and add it to the fish with the onion. Add the seeds, the chicken seasoning and the wine and mix. Reduce heat.

- Let it boil for a minute or two and pour the almonds into a small, heavy fish, remaining in a tablespoon of butter. When the almonds are golden, pour them into the rice and serve.

- Yield: 5 servings

- Each with 4 grams of carbohydrates and 1 gram of fiber, for a total of 3 grams of usable carbohydrates and 2 grams of protein

# Raspberry Chia Breakfast Jars

**Ingredients**

- 12 ounces (340 g) frozen raspberries, thawed but not drained
- 12 ounces (340 g) soft silken tofu or unsweetened plain vegan yogurt
- ¼ cup (80 g) pure maple syrup
- 2 tablespoons (24 g) maple sugar or (30 g) light brown sugar, optional
- ¼ cup (48 g) white chia seeds
- ¼ teaspoon pure vanilla extract

- 6 ounces (170 g) fresh berries (raspberries or blueberries), rinsed and thoroughly drained

**Instructions**

- Place the melted raspberries in the blender or use a submerged blender to mix the berries. If you don't like blackberries, pass this mixture through a fine mesh sieve. Add tofu or yogurt, maple syrup and sugar to the berries and mix again to mix. Put in a large bowl.
- Mix the chia seeds and vanilla in the mixture. Cover and refrigerate for at least 3 hours or overnight. Stir before serving.
- Place some fresh berries in the bottom of the jar. (You can also mix the berries directly in the mixture and keep some to season).
- Divide the chia preparation on top and sprinkle with the berries.
- Remaining can be stored in an airtight container in the refrigerator for up to 4 days.

**Yield**:

6 servings

**Protein content per serving:**

7 g

# Venetian "Rice"

## Ingredients

- ½ head cauliflower
- 1 tablespoon (15 ml) olive oil
- 2 tablespoons (28 g) butter
- 1 cup (100 g) sliced mushrooms
- 3 anchovy fillets, minced
- 1 clove garlic, crushed
- 3 tablespoons (18.8 g) grated Parmesan cheese

## Instructions

- Run cauliflower through the food processor chopper. Put it in a microwave-safe bowl with a lid, add a few tablespoons (30 ml) of water, cover and simmer for 5 to 6 minutes.

- When you're done, discover it right away! Combine olive oil and butter in a large, heavy skillet over medium heat and mix until well combined.

- Add mushrooms and sauces to make the color soft and changeable. If the slices of mushrooms are large enough, you may want to break the edge of the spatula slightly when slicing.

- When the mushrooms are soft, beat in the pan and stir. Add rice and brown without eggs - which will help a little water to mix. Mix well to distribute all the flavors.
- Stir in the parmesan and serve.
- Yield: 3 to 4 servings
- Each will have 4 grams of protein. 2 grams of carbohydrates; 1 gram of dietary fiber; 1 gram of usable carbon.

# Blackened Mexican Tofu, Greens, and Hash Browns

### Ingredients

- 2 teaspoons onion powder
- Preheat the oven to 300°F
- 2 teaspoons chipotle chili powder
- 1 teaspoon garlic powder
- 1 teaspoon smoked paprika
- 1 teaspoon dried oregano, crushed to a powder using fingers
- ½ teaspoon fine sea salt

- 1 pound (454 g) extra-firm tofu, drained, pressed, and cut into ½-inch (1.3 cm) slices
- 1 tablespoon (15 ml) high heat neutral-flavored oil
- 2 bunches (1½ pounds, or 681 g) Swiss chard, chopped
- 2 tablespoons (15 g) nutritional yeast
- 1 package (1 pound, or 454 g) hash browns
- 1 avocado, pitted, peeled, and sliced Salsa, for serving

**Instructions**

- Combine the onion powder, chili powder, garlic powder, smoked paprika, oregano, and salt on a plate. Coat the tofu with the spice mixture. Heat the oil in a large skillet over high heat. Test the heat of the oil by dipping a corner of tofu into it. It should sizzle. Cook the tofu slices for 3 to 5 minutes until blackened. Turn over to cook the second side for 3 to 4 minutes until also blackened. Keep warm in the oven.

- Reduce the heat to medium. Put the Swiss chard into the same skillet. If the Swiss chard is freshly washed, it will still be slightly wet. If not. add a tablespoon (15 ml) of water, if needed, so it doesn't stick. Add the nutritional yeast and cook for 4 to 6 minutes, stirring occasionally, until wilted.

- To serve, place one-quarter of the Swiss chard on each plate. Top with one-quarter of the hash browns and 2 to 3 pieces of tofu, depending on how many slices you were able to get. Place a few slices of avocado on the plate and serve the salsa on the side.

**Yield:**

4 servings

**Protein Content Per Serving:**

18 g

# Smoky Bean and Tempeh Patties

**Ingredients**

- 1 cup (177 g) cooked cannellini beans
- 8 ounces (227 g) tempeh
- ½ cup (91 g) cooked bulgur
- 2 cloves garlic, pressed
- 1½ teaspoons onion powder
- 4 teaspoons (20 ml) liquid smoke
- 4 teaspoons (20 ml) Worcestershire sauce
- 1 teaspoon smoked paprika
- 2 tablespoons (30 g) organic ketchup
- 2 tablespoons (40 g) pure maple syrup

- 2 tablespoons (30 ml) neutral- flavored oil
- 3 tablespoons (45 ml) tamari
- ½ cup (60 g) chickpea flour
- Nonstick cooking spray

**Instructions**

Mash the beans in a large bowl: It's okay if a few small pieces of beans are left. Crumble (do not mash) the tempeh into small pieces on top. Add the bulgur and garlic. In a medium bowl, whisk together the remaining ingredients, except the flour and cooking spray. Stir into the crumbled tempeh preparation. Add the flour and mix until well combined. Chill for 1 hour before shaping into patties.

Preheat the oven to 350°F (180°C, or gas mark 4). Line a baking sheet with parchment paper. Scoop out a packed ½ cup (96 g) per patty, shaping into an approximately 3-inch (8 cm) circle and flattening slightly on the prepared sheet. You should get eight 3.5-inch (9 cm) patties in all. Lightly coat the top of the patties with cooking spray. Bake for 15 minutes, carefully flip, lightly coat the top of the patties with cooking spray, and bake for another 15 minutes until lightly browned and firm.

Leftovers can be stored in an airtight container in the refrigerator for up to 4 days. The patties can also be frozen, tightly wrapped in foil, for up to 3 months.

If you don't eat all the patties at once, reheat the leftovers on low heat in a skillet lightly greased with olive oil or cooking spray for about 5 minutes on each side until heated through.

**Yield:**

8 patties

**Protein Content Per Patty:**

10 g

# Nuts and Seeds Breakfast Cookies

## Ingredients

- 6 tablespoons (72 g) Sucanat
- 2 tablespoons (40 g) pure maple syrup
- ¼ cup (60 g) blended soft silken tofu or vanilla vegan yogurt
- ¼ cup (64 g) natural creamy cashew butter
- 2 tablespoons (30 ml) neutral-flavored oil
- ¼ teaspoon pure vanilla extract
- Scant ¼ teaspoon fine sea salt
- ¼ teaspoon ginger powder or ground cinnamon
- ¼ cup (15 g) freeze-dried raspberries
- 3 tablespoons (30 g) shelled hemp seeds

- 1¼ cups (120 g) old-fashioned oats
- ¼ cup (90 g) whole wheat pastry flour
- ¼ teaspoon baking powder

**Instructions**

- Preheat oven to 350°F (180°C, or gas mark 4). Line a large cookie sheet with parchment paper or a silicone baking mat.
- In a large mixing bowl, combine the Sucanat, maple syrup, yogurt or tofu, cashew butter, oil, vanilla, salt, and ginger powder.
- Add the berries, seeds, and oats on top. Sift the flour and baking powder on top.
- Stir until well combined. Let stand for 5 minutes.
- Scoop a packed ¼ cup (about 60 g) of dough per cookie onto the prepared sheet. Flatten slightly because the cookies won't spread a lot while baking. Repeat with the remaining 7 cookies.
- Bake for 14 minutes or until the edges of the cookies are a light golden brown. Let cool on the sheet for 5 minutes before transferring to a cooling rack.
- These are best served still warm from the oven or at room temperature. Store leftovers in an airtight container for up to 2 days.

**Yield:**

8 big cookies

**Protein content per serving:**

5 g

# Japanese Fried "Rice"

## Ingredients

- ½ head cauliflower, shredded
- 2 eggs
- 1 cup (75 g) snow pea pods, fresh
- 2 tablespoons (28 g) butter
- ½ cup (80 g) diced onion
- 2 tablespoons (16 g) shredded carrot
- 3 tablespoons (45 ml) soy sauce Salt and pepper

## Instructions

- With a microwave lid, add a few tablespoons (30 ml) of water, cover the microwave for 6 minutes.
- While this is happening, beat the eggs, pour into a non-stick cooking pan and cook over medium-high heat. When you cook the eggs, use your spatulas to chop the size of the egg. Separate yourself from specialists and set aside.

- Remove the peas and rows of snow peas and draw an inch (6 mm) long. (The microwave is already humming. Remove it from the cauliflower or turn it into a mushroom that doesn't look like rice at all!)

- Melt the butter in a pan and leave the peas, onions and carrots for 2 to 3 minutes. Add cauliflower and mix well. Stir in the soy sauce and cook all the ingredients, stirring frequently for another 5-6 minutes. Add some salt and pepper and serve.

**Yield:**

5 servings

Each with 4 grams of protein; 5 grams of carbohydrates; 1 gram of dietary fiber; 4 grams of carbohydrates.

## Tilapia on a Nest of Vegetables

**Ingredients**

- 1-pound (455 g) tilapia fillets
- 3 tablespoons (45 ml) olive oil
- 1 cup (150 g) red pepper, cut into thin strips
- 1 cup (150 g) yellow pepper, cut into thin strips
- 1½ cups (180 g) zucchini, cut in matchstick strips
- 1½ cups (180 g) yellow squash, cut in matchstick strips

- 1 cup (160 g) sweet red onion, thinly sliced
- 1 clove garlic, crushed
- Salt and pepper
- ¼ teaspoon guar or xanthan
- Lemon wedges (optional)

**Instructions**

- Heat the olive oil in a heavy skillet over medium heat and leave the peppers, pumpkins, pumpkins, onions and garlic just 2 to 3 minutes and stir constantly.
- Sprinkle the tilapia fillets with salt and pepper on both sides, then place the vegetables in the pan. Cover, heat slightly over medium heat and allow the fish to evaporate in the vegetable moisture for 10 minutes or until lightly crusted.
- Using a slice, carefully transfer the fish to a serving plate and use a spoon to collect the vegetables over the fish. Pour liquid into the pan in the mixer and add guar or xanthan. Run the mixer for a few seconds and then pour the concentrated water over the fish and vegetables. To serve, place a slice of vegetables on a plate on each table and place a slice of fish on it. Some lemon wedges are good in this regard, but hardly necessary.

**Yield:**

4 servings

Each has 11 grams of carbohydrates and 2 grams of fiber, for a total of 8 grams of carbohydrates and 22 grams of protein.

# Balsamic-Mustard Chicken

## Ingredients

- 1 broiler-fryer chicken, about 3 pounds (1.4 kg), cut up, or whatever chicken parts you like
- 2 tablespoons (33 g) chili garlic paste
- ½ cup (120 ml) spicy brown mustard
- ¼ cup (60 ml) balsamic vinegar ¼ cup (60 ml) olive oil

## Instructions

- Put the chicken pieces in a large heavy plastic bag. Combine everything else and hit it together. Reserve a little marinade to lean on and then chop the rest with the chicken, squeeze the air and seal the bag. Pour the bag into the refrigerator and allow the chicken to marinate hourly all day.
- When it's time to cook, turn on your coal or gas stove. You want a medium to medium fire. When the oven is ready, remove the chicken from the marinade using a tong and place it on a plate. Pour the marinade.

- Now place the chicken on the grill skin and fry for 12 to 15 minutes. Turn it around and allow it to brown 7 to 9 minutes on one side of the skin. Turn it over and bake for another 5 to 10 minutes or read 180 degrees Fahrenheit (85 degrees Celsius) until the water clears when the bone is pierced and reads an instant thermometer. Repeat with the reserved marinade once again using clean dishes each time you eat. Keep the grill closed, unless you cook or turn the chicken.

**Yield:**

5 to 6 servings

Assume 6 servings, if you have consumed all the marinade, each has 3 grams of carbohydrates and fiber, but you will actually get less. Assuming 6 servings, each will contain 30 grams of protein

## Lonestar "Rice"

**Ingredients**

- ½ head cauliflower, shredded
- 1 tablespoon (15 ml) olive oil
- 1 tablespoon (14 g) butter
- ¼ cup (40 g) chopped onion
- 1 cup (100 g) sliced mushrooms

- ½ cup (40 g) snow pea pods, fresh, cut in ½-inch (1.3-cm) pieces
- ¼ teaspoon chili powder
- 2 teaspoons beef bouillon granules or concentrate

**Instructions**

- Put cauliflower with a lid in the microwave oven. Add 6 tablespoons (30 ml) of water, cover and microwave for 6 minutes.
- While cooking, heat the olive oil and butter in a large fish and smooth the onion, mushrooms and snow peas. I like to use the edge of the spatula to cut the mushrooms into smaller pieces, but if you like the way you cut them better - it's up to you.
- When the mushrooms have changed and the snow pea is completely clear, drain the cooked rice and add it in the pepper and beef powder, mix to distribute the seasonings and then serve.

**Yield:**

3 servings

Each has 2 grams of protein; 5 grams of carbohydrates; 1 gram of dietary fiber; 4 grams of carbohydrates.

Lunch

# Quick & Easy Tomato and Herb Gigantes Beans

**Ingredients**

- 2 tbsp. olive oil
- 1 onion
- 1 carrot
- 1 tsp ready-chopped garlic Protein content per serving garlic purée
- 1 Protein content per serving2 tsp paprika
- 400 g tin butterbeans
- 400 g tin chopped tomatoes
- 2 tbsp. tomato purée
- 1 tsp sugar
- 2 tsp dried oregano
- handful baby spinach
- handful fresh parsley
- 8-10 fresh mint leaves

## Instructions

Heat the oil in a large pot or in a large pot with oil. Chop onions and carrots and chop them finely and add them to the pot with garlic and paprika. Cook over medium heat for 2 minutes.

Rinse and wash the potatoes and add to the pot, then add the greased tomatoes. Fill the empty tomato can in half with water and add it to the pot with tomato puree, sugar and oregano. Season well with salt and black pepper, boil, then reduce at dawn, cover and cook for 12-14 minutes.

Chop the baby spinach approximately, then add them to the pot and cook for 2 minutes. Chop the parsley and mint almost and stir just before serving. Taste and adjust the seasoning if necessary, then serve with crusty bread and crispy green salad.

## Yield:

2 Servings

# Chinese Sticky Wings

## Ingredients

- 3 pounds (1.4 kg) chicken wings
- ¼ cup (60 ml) dry sherry
- ¼ cup (60 ml) soy sauce

- ¼ cup (60 ml) sugar-free imitation honey
- 1 tablespoon (6 g) grated ginger root
- 1 clove garlic
- ½ teaspoon chili garlic paste

**Instructions**

- If complete, cut the wings to "resistance". Put the wings in a large plastic bag that can be used.
- Mix everything else and reserve a little marinade to loosen and pour the rest into the bag. Seal the bag and press the air as you go. Turn the bag several times to cover the wings and chill in the refrigerator for several hours (a whole day is bright).
- Preheat the oven to 375 degrees Fahrenheit (190 degrees Celsius or marked gas 5). Pull the bag, pour the marinade and place the wings on a shallow plate and allow them to cook for one hour in the oven, then marinate every 15 minutes. Use a clean container every time you eat.
- Serve with lots of napkins!
- Yield: Approximately 28 pieces
- Each with 5 grams of protein; carbohydrate tracking; dietary fiber Tracking usable carbohydrates Carbon numbers do not include honey-free mimicry.

# Pappardelle with Cavolo Nero & Walnut Sauce

**Yield:**

2 Servings

**Ingredients**

- 200 g cavolo nero
- 150 g walnut pieces
- 250 g Pappardelle pasta linguine
- 1 slice bread
- 150 g dairy-free milk (soya, oat or nut milk)
- 2 tbsp. fresh parsley
- optional - 2 tbsp. vegan parmesan or nutritional yeast flakes
- 1 clove garlic
- olive oil

**Instructions**

- Remove the kale stems and cut them into slices of protein per serving.

- Heat a pan, peel the nuts (no oil needed) and bake over medium heat for 2-3 minutes. Turn off the heat and reserve.

- Boil a large pot of water and soak Caverno Nero for 1 minute, then use a slotted spoon or tweezers to remove it and remove it with a sieve or stain (remove the boiling water in the pot).

- Add the papardel to the boiling water and simmer for 8-10 minutes.

- Meanwhile, sprinkle nuts, bread, milk protein content in each serving of milk, parsley, garlic and Parmesan (if used) in a blender or food mixture and mix until consistent. Reach the thick sauce, beat it. Season well with salt and black pepper.

- Heat the pan again, add a little olive oil and put it in Kawlow Norway. Cook for 3-4 minutes and turn off the heat.

- When the pasta is cooked, drain it and return it to the pot. Tilt and add the walnut sauce to combine. Finally, add caolo nero, overlay and then divide between two dishes.

# Wicked Wings

### Ingredeiants

- 4 pounds (1.8 kg) chicken wings
- 1 cup (100 g) grated Parmesan cheese

- 2 tablespoons (2.6 g) dried parsley
- 1 tablespoon (5.4 g) dried oregano
- 2 teaspoons paprika 1 teaspoon salt
- ½ teaspoon pepper ½ cup butter

**Instructions**

- Heat the oven to 350 degrees F (180 degrees Celsius or gas 4). Line a shallow pan with foil. (Do not miss this step or clean the pan a week later.)
- Saving interesting things, cut the wings into "sticks". (Not sure what to do with wing tips? Freeze them for soup. Have a good broth.)
- Combine parmesan and parsley, oregano, pepper, salt and pepper in a bowl.
- Melt the butter in a shallow bowl or pan
- Soak each roast in butter, roll in cheese and spice mixture and place in lined pan.
- Bake for 1-hour B and then beat to avoid making a double recipe!
- Yield: About 50 pieces
- Each has only carbohydrates, fiber and 4 grams of protein.

# Veggie Sausage & Sun-Dried Tomato One Pot Pasta

**Yield:**

4 Servings

**Ingredients**

- 2 tbsp. olive or rapeseed oil
- 3 veggie sausages
- 1 onion, peeled and sliced
- 400 g pasta shells
- 200 g cherry tomatoes, halved
- 6-8 sun-dried tomatoes, roughly chopped
- 1-liter water
- 2 tsp vegetable stock powder
- 100 ml dairy-free cream (I used soya)
- 100 g fresh baby spinach

**Instructions**

- Heat the oil in a large, shallow dish and fry the sausage and onion until the sausages brown. Carefully separate them from the pan and cut each piece into slices into 4 pieces, then return to the pot for another 2 minutes.

- Add pasta, tomatoes, sun-dried tomatoes, water and powder to the pot. Bring to a boil, then reduce to a sweet boil, cover and cook for 12-14 minutes, stirring every few minutes, until the pasta is well cooked.

- Add the cream and spinach to the pot, then stir well and cook for another minute until the spinach has vanished.

## Roast Chicken with Balsamic Vinegar

### Ingredients

- 1 cut up broiler-fryer Bay Leaves Salt or Vege-Sal Pepper
- 3 to 4 tablespoons (45 to 60 ml) olive oil
- 3 to 4 tablespoons (42 to 56 g) butter
- ½ cup (60 ml) dry white wine 3 tablespoons (45 ml) balsamic vinegar
- Preheat the oven to 350°F (180°C, or gas mark 4).

### Instructions

- Wrap a sheet or two of leaves under the skin of each slice of chicken and sprinkle each slice with salt and pepper and place them in the grill pan.

- Soak the chicken with olive oil and cover with the same butter. Roast in the oven for 1 V2 hours and rotate each piece every 20 to 30 minutes. (This makes the skin gloriously crisp and pleasant.)

- When the chicken is ready, place it on a plate and pour the fat from the pan. Put the pan over medium heat and pour the wine and balsamic vinegar. Mix this loop and dissolve the delicious sweets that are glued in the cooking pan. Boil this in just a minute or two, pour into a pot or jar and serve with chicken. Throw in bay leaves before serving.

**Yield:**

4 servings

Each contains 2 grams of carbohydrates, fiber and 44 grams of protein

# Orange-Five-Spice Roasted Chicken

**Ingredients**

- 3 pounds (1.4 kg) chicken thighs
- ¼ cup (60 ml) soy sauce
- 2 tablespoons (30 ml) canola or peanut oil
- 1 tablespoon (15 ml) lemon juice
- 1 tablespoon (15 ml) white wine vinegar

- 1 tablespoon (1.5 g) Splenda
- 2 tablespoons (40 g) low-sugar orange marmalade
- 2 teaspoons five-spice powder

**Instructions**

- Put the chicken in a large plastic bag. Mix everything together. Reserve a little marinade for weight loss and pour the rest into the bag. Seal the bag and press the air as you go. Turn the bag over to cover the chicken and place it in the refrigerator. Allow for at least two hours and this is a good time.
- Heat the oven to 375 degrees Fahrenheit (190 degrees Celsius). Remove the chicken from the refrigerator, pour the marinade and place the chicken in a pan and fry the chicken for 1 hour.
- Reserved with Marinade 2 or 3 times, be sure to use clean containers every time you eat to avoid cross contamination.

**Yield:**

5 to 6 servings

Assuming each will have 32 grams of protein.

3 grams of carbohydrates; dietary fiber tracking 3 grams of usable carbohydrates - and you're supposed to consume whole marinade.

# Microwaved Fish and Asparagus with Tarragon Mustard Sauce

## Ingredients

- 12 ounces (340 g) fish fillets— whiting, tilapia, sole, flounder, or any kind of white fish
- 10 asparagus spears
- 2 tablespoons (30 g) sour cream
- 1 tablespoon (15 g) mayonnaise
- ¼ teaspoon dried tarragon
- ½ teaspoon Dijon or spicy brown mustard

## Instructions

- Draw the bottom of the asparagus spears and cut them naturally. Put the asparagus on a large glass plate, add 1 teaspoon (15 ml) of water and cover with a plate. Microwave for 3 minutes.
- While the asparagus is in the microwave, mix sour, mayonnaise, tarragon and mustard together.
- Remove the asparagus from the microwave oven, remove it from the pie plate and set aside. Drain the water from the runway. Put the fish fillet in it

- Peel the pie plate and spread 2 tablespoons (30 ml) cream mixture on them and cover the pie again and place the fish in the microwave for 3 to 4 minutes. Open the oven, remove the plate from the top of the pie plate and place the asparagus on top of the fish. Cover the pie plate again and cook for another 1-2 minutes.

- Remove the pie plate from the microwave oven and remove the plate. Put the fish and asparagus on a serving platter. Chop any boiled sauce on a plate over fish and asparagus. Melt each with reserved sauce and serve.

- Yield: 2 servings

- Each with 4 grams of carbohydrates and 2 grams of fiber, for a total of 2 grams of usable carbohydrates and 33 grams of protein

- It also packs 949 mg of potassium!

## Orange-Tangerine Up-the- Butt Chicken

**Ingredients**

- 3½ to 4-pound (1.6 to 1.8 kg) whole roasting chicken
- 1 teaspoon salt or Vege-Sal
- 1 teaspoon Splenda

- 1 drop blackstrap molasses (It helps to keep your molasses in a squeeze bottle.)
- 1 teaspoon chili powder
- 3 tablespoons (60 g) low-sugar orange marmalade
- 1 12-ounce (360-ml) can tangerine Diet-Rite soda, divided (Make sure the can is clean!)
- 2 to 3 teaspoons oil
- 1 teaspoon spicy brown mustard

**Instructions**

- Prepare your grill for indirect cooking - if you have a gas stove, just light it on one side. If using charcoal, place the lighter on one side of the grill and light.
- Remove the chicken's neck and towels and wash the chicken and dry it with paper towels.
- In a small bowl of salt or Vege-Sal, mix Splenda, molasses and red pepper powder. Pour half of the mixture (1/8 teaspoon) into a bowl and store. Rub the rest into the chicken hole.
- Mix the orange marmalade with low sugar in the reserved spice mixture. Open the tangerine boxes and pour 3.2 cups (160 ml). Put N cup (60 ml) of the beverage in a jam / spice mixture and mix - you can drain or throw away the remaining siphon you

poured. Now, using a church-style console door, pull several holes at the top of the can. Cover the box with non-stick cooking spray and place it in a deep bowl. Carefully place the chicken on the boxes and place the can inside the chicken cavity. Rub the chicken with oil.

- Okay, you're ready to cook! Make sure you place a pan. Set the chicken to rotate vertically on the beverage cans on the side of the oven, not above the fire and gently spread the drums to create a tripod effect. Close the grill and cook the chicken at 250 degrees Fahrenheit (130 degrees Celsius) or about 75 to 90 minutes or until the juices are clear when the bone sticks. You can also use a meat thermometer. Must have 180 degrees Fahrenheit (85 degrees Celsius).

- While the chicken is cooking, add the mustard to the jam / soda / spice mixture and mix all the ingredients. Use this mixture for the chicken dough for the last 20 minutes or fry.

- When the chicken is finished, carefully separate it from the grill. Grill gloves are useful here or use hot pads and piles. Wrap the tins and separate them from the chicken and discard. Allow the chicken to rest for 5 minutes before sculpting. Meanwhile, heat each remaining sweetened sauce until boiling and serve as chicken sauce.

**Yield:**

5 servings

Each serving contains 5 grams of carbohydrates and one trace of fiber. Assuming a chicken weighs 2.3 kilograms (1.6 kg), each serving will have 40 grams of protein.

# Almond-Stuffed Flounder Rolls with Orange Butter Sauce

**Ingredients**

- 1 pound (455 g) flounder fillets, 4 ounces (115 g) each
- 4 tablespoons (56 g) butter, divided
- 2 tablespoons (30 ml) lemon juice
- 1/8 teaspoon orange extract
- 1 teaspoon Splenda
- ½ cup (45 g) almonds
- ¼ cup (40 g) minced onion
- 1 clove garlic, crushed
- 1½ teaspoons Dijon mustard
- ½ teaspoon soy sauce
- ¼ cup (15.2 g) minced fresh parsley, divided

## Instructions

- 2 tablespoons (28 g) butter, lemon juice, orange juice and splendor in a slow cooker. Cover the slow cooker, lower it and allow it to warm up as you secure the circular bearings.

- Place the almonds in a food mixture and chop them into a cornstarch. 1 tablespoon butter (14 g), melt the butter in a medium bowl and add the almonds. Bake almonds over medium heat for 5 to 7 minutes or until fragrant. Transfer them to a bowl.

- Now melt the final spoon (14 g) of butter in a pan and boil the onion and garlic over medium-low heat until the onion is clear. Add them to the almonds and mix. Now mix the mustard, soy sauce and 2 teaspoons (7.6 g) of parsley.

- Wrap the wool fillets on a large plate and divide the almond mixture between them and wrap it over the fillets, then glue them together and glue them with a toothpick.

- Remove the lid from the slow cooker and mix the sauce. Put the rolls in the sauce and spoon the sauce over them. Cover the dish again and let it cook for 1 hour. When you are done, place the sauce on them and sprinkle the parsley left on it for serving.

## Return:

4 servings

Each has 24 grams of protein, 5 grams of carbohydrates, 2 grams of dietary fiber, 3 grams of carbohydrates.

# Sherry-Mustard-Soy Marinated Chicken

**Ingredients**

- 3 ½ to 4 pounds (1.6 to 1.8 kg) cut-up chicken
- ¼ cup (6 g) Splenda
- 3 tablespoons (45 ml) olive oil
- 3 tablespoons (45 ml) sherry
- 1 tablespoon (15 ml) mustard
- 1 tablespoon (15 ml) soy sauce
- 1 tablespoon (6.3 g) black pepper
- ½ tablespoon Worcestershire sauce
- ¼ cup (40 g) minced onion
- 1 clove garlic, crushed
- 2 tablespoons (30 ml) water

**Instructions**

- Mix everything, except the chicken, mix well. Put the chicken in a shallow pan, without reaction, or in a plastic bag. Reserve a little marinade to be weak and pour the remaining marinade over the chicken. If it is in a vessel, close it once or twice to cover it. If it is in a bag, remove the air, seal the bag and rotate it several times to cover the chicken. In any case, wrap the chicken in the refrigerator and let it boil for at least 1 or 2 hours and not be injured.

- When the chicken is ready for the oven, place the oven on medium charcoal or charcoal covered with white ash. Rinse the chicken bone with the lid closed for 10 to 12 minutes (but check the flames from time to time!) And with the marinade reserved once or twice using a clean container, each time you cook, you lean. Turn the chicken loose and fry it on the skin for 6 to 7 minutes, then grate again, but now and then check to make it go away. Start the chicken in the bone, soak it again and grill with the lid closed for another 5 to 10 minutes until the water when the chicken water is cleaned of the bone when the chicken is pierced or until a thermometer reads 180 immediately. Delete it. Fahrenheit (85 ° C).

**Yield:**

5 to 6 servings

Suppose 6 and assume the consumption of whole marinade, each serving of 4 grams of carbohydrates and 1 gram of fiber, is 3 grams usable for the number of carbohydrates. However, since you will not eat all the marinade, I count 2 grams per serving. 34 grams of protein.

# Two-Cheese Tuna-Stuffed Mushrooms

## Ingredients

- ½ pound (225 g) fresh mushrooms
- 1 can (6 ounces, or 170 g) tuna
- ½ cup (60 g) shredded smoked Gouda
- 2 tablespoons (12.5 g) grated Parmesan cheese
- 3 tablespoons (42 g) mayonnaise 1 scallion, finely minced

## Instructions

- Heat the oven to 350 degrees F (180 degrees Celsius or gas 4).
- Clean the mushrooms with a damp cloth and remove the stems.
- Barbecue tuna, gouda, parmesan, mayonnaise and onion
- Mix well.
- Pour the mixture into the mushroom covers and place in a shallow frying pan, add just enough water to cover the pan, cook for 15 minutes and serve hot.

## Yield:

approximately 15 servings

Each contains 1 gram of carbohydrates, one trace of fiber and 4 grams of protein.

**Dinner**

# Cauliflower Rice Deluxe

## Ingredients

- 3 cups (500 g) cauliflower rice— about ½ head's worth
- ¼ cup (50 g) wild rice
- ¼ cup (180 ml) water

## Instructions

Make your own cauliflower rice as you want - Prepare the microwave oven so be careful not to put it on the mushroom. You want to bid. Pour rice and wild water into a bowl, cover and simmer until all the water is gone - at least half an hour, maybe a little longer. Cook cauliflower rice and mix in the wild rice and season as desired.

## Yield:

8 servings

Even with wild rice, it has only 6 grams of carbohydrates, with 1 gram of fiber, for 5 grams of carbohydrates per cup (85 grams).

# Creamy Wild Mushroom One-Pot Gnocchi

**Yield:**

2 Servings

**Protein Content Per Servings:**

13.5 g

**Ingredients**

- 5 small shallots
- 2 tbsp. rapeseed or olive oil
- 1 tsp ready-chopped garlic
- 250 g mixed mushrooms
- 500 g ready-made gnocchi
- 125 ml white wine
- 125 ml vegetable stock
- handful baby spinach
- 3 tbsp. soya cream
- vegan parmesan-style 'cheese' (optional)

## Instructions

Peel the shells and chop them finely. Soak the oil in a large pan or large saucepan and simmer for 2-3 minutes and soak the crumbs and garlic until soft.

Chop or halve the mushrooms (depending on their size) and add them to the pot. Turn on the heat and cook for 3-4 minutes to keep the water free. Season well with salt and black pepper.

Add the gnocchi and then the white wine and let it bubble for a minute, then pour over the vegetables, return to a medium blender, cover with a lid and cook for 5 minutes, stirring occasionally.

Chop the spinach almost, then stir, followed by the soy cream. Adjust seasoning if necessary and adjust if necessary, then serve immediately with a piece of vegan parmesan.

# Black Bean & Avocado Tacos

**Yield:**

2 Servings

**Ingredients**

- 1 tbsp. rapeseed or sunflower oil
- half a red onion

- 1 tsp ready-chopped garlic or garlic puree
- 200 g tinned black beans
- 5 cherry tomatoes
- 1 roasted red pepper
- half an avocado
- juice of half a lime
- handful fresh coriander
- 2 tortilla wraps

**Instructions**

- Heat the oil in a small pan. Peel and chop the onion and add to the pot and then the garlic. Cook for 2 minutes. Wash and wash black beans and put them inside. Mix well with salt and black pepper and cook over medium heat for another 3-4 minutes, stirring occasionally.

- Meanwhile, cut the cherry tomatoes in half and chop the peppers into thin strips. Remove the stone from the avocado and cut it into 1 cm pieces. Combine the tomatoes, peppers and avocado in a small bowl and season with salt and black pepper. Press the lemon juice and pour everything into the mixture.

- Heat a second pan and lightly brown the sides of the cream until lightly browned.

- Chop the coriander leaves almost and mix them with the tomato and avocado mixture.

- Place the roasted tortillas in layers with beans and onions, then mix the tomatoes, peppers and avocado and serve immediately.

# Spatchcocked or UnSpatchcocked Chicken with Vinegar Baste

## Ingredients

- 3 ½ pounds (1.6 kg) chicken— either whole or cut up
- 1 cup (240 ml) cider vinegar 3 teaspoons chili powder
- 2 tablespoons (3 g) Splenda
- 1 teaspoon cayenne 1 teaspoon paprika
- 1 teaspoon dry mustard 1 teaspoon black pepper ½ teaspoon cumin ½ teaspoon salt

## Instructions

- Technically, you'll have to cut both sides of the spine and remove it completely, but that's too much for me, so I'll just leave my baby.

- You look rough, I know it sounds hard, but if you have chicken or kitchen scissors - my Marta Stewart scissors are great at Kmart

- it all takes about a minute and a half Along the bottom of the chicken, grab each one. Open the cut and the chicken and press on the bones to hear a slight gap. Now you have a flat chicken that you can place on the grill.

- Or you just can't be bothered. Describe this process because it is very interesting, very trendy right now, and yet whole chickens are often very cheap. However, I think using chopped chicken is easier, you know? These wastes work well with parts and do not have to be carved.

- However, start to start the stove. You want it over medium heat. While the oven is warming, mix everything except the chicken.

- Grill the chicken that started from the skin and keep the grill closed, except those with frost or flame, for 15 minutes and each time using a vinegar mixture. Clean, liquid. Turn some of the skin down and fry for 7 to 9 minutes, still boring. Then pull the skin back on and continue to grill to clean the water when the chicken is pierced or record a thermometer reading 180 degrees Fahrenheit (85 degrees Celsius). Service.

**Yield:**

5 servings

Even with all the boiled liquid, you will only get 5 grams of carbohydrates, 1 gram of fiber or 4 grams of carbohydrate per serving

- but you will not consume all the nutrients. Count over 2 grams per serving. 40 grams of protein.

## Pan-Barbecued Sea Bass

### Ingredients

- 1-pound (455 g) sea bass fillets
- 1 tablespoon (8 g) Classic Barbecue Rub
- 4 slices bacon
- 2 tablespoons (30 ml) lemon juice

### Instructions

- Cut the sea bass fillets into pieces. Sprinkle both sides freely with a grill.
- Grease a large, heavy fish with nonstick cooking spray and cook over medium-low heat. Using sharp kitchen scissors, pour the bacon into small pieces directly into a fisherman. Shake it for a moment. As soon as you start cooking some fat from the bacon, wipe out a pair of fish and place the fish in the pan. Cover and set the oven timer for 4 minutes.
- When the time is up, cook the fish and mix a little bacon to make it even. Restore the vessel and set the stopwatch for another 3-

4 minutes. Look at your fish at least once. You don't want to overtake him!

- When the fish has collapsed, you should serve the dishes and add the brown bacon. Pour lemon juice into the pan, mix and pour over the fish. Service.

**Yield:**

3 servings

Each with 31 grams of protein; 2 grams of carbohydrates; dietary fiber tracking 2 grams of carbohydrates.

# Absolutely Classic Barbecued Chicken

## Ingredients

- 3 pounds (1.4 kg) cut-up chicken (on the bone, skin on—choose light or dark meat, as you prefer)
- 1 ½ cup (40 g) Classic Barbecue Rub
- ½ cup (120 ml) chicken broth
- ½ cup (120 ml) oil
- ½ cup (120 ml) Kansas City Barbecue Sauce

## Instructions

- The chips or pieces of wood are softened for at least 30 minutes

- Continue with the grill and set it for indirect smoking.
- While the oven is warming, sprinkle the chicken with a spoon
- Scrub Combine reserved scrub with broth and chicken oil to combine.
- When the fire is ready, place the chicken on a greased pan, add wood chips or slices and close the grill. Let him smoke half an hour before you start smoking.
- Then, each time you use a chip or more pieces, use a clean container each time you use it.
- Smoke the chicken approximately 90 minutes or until an instant thermometer reads 180 degrees Fahrenheit (85 degrees Celsius).
- When the chicken is finished, soak the skin in a Kansas City barbecue sauce and let it simmer for 5 minutes or on the fire near the skin.
- Rinse the other side with the sauce using a clean bowl, wrap it and put on the heat for another 5 minutes.
- Boil the remaining sauce and serve with chicken
- Avoid this same basic method using any type of scrub and any sauce!

**Yield:**

5 servings

For each serving of 9 grams of carbohydrates and 1 gram of fiber, there are 8 grams of usable carbohydrates. 35 grams of protein.

# Company Dinner "Rice"

## Ingredients

- 1 small onion, chopped
- 1 stick (115 g) butter, melted
- 1 batch Cauliflower Rice Deluxe
- 6 strips bacon, cooked until crisp, and crumbled
- ¼ teaspoon salt or Vege-Sal
- ¼ teaspoon pepper
- ½ cup (50 g) grated Parmesan cheese

## Instructions

Sprinkle the onion in butter until golden and brown. Cauliflower Delicious luxury cauliflower with onion and shaved bacon, salt, pepper and cheese. Service.

## Yield:

8 servings

Each with 8 grams of carbohydrates and 2 grams of fiber, for a total of 6 grams of usable carbohydrates and 5 grams of protein.

# Soy and Ginger Pecans

## Ingredients

- 2 cups (200 g) shelled pecans
- 4 tablespoons (56 g) butter, melted
- 3 tablespoons (45 ml) soy sauce
- 1 teaspoon ground ginger

## Instructions

- Heat the oven to 300 degrees Fahrenheit (150 degrees Celsius or gas 2).
- Sprinkle the muffins in a shallow frying pan and shake the butter and cover all the nuts.
- Roast for 15 minutes, then remove from the oven and stir in the soy sauce. Sprinkle the ginger evenly over the walnut and mix.
- Roast for another 10 minutes.

## Yield:

8 servings

Each 6 grams of carbohydrates and 2 grams of fiber, for a total of 4 grams of usable carbohydrates and 3 grams of protein.

# Hearty Quinoa Waffles

**Yield:**

6 to 8 waffles

**Protein Content Per Waffle:**

7 g

**Ingredients**

- 1½ cups (355 ml) water, divided
- ⅔ cup (119 g) chopped dates
- 3 tablespoons (42 g) solid coconut oil
- 3 tablespoons (60 g) pure maple syrup
- 1½ teaspoons pure vanilla extract
- 1¾ cups (210 g) whole wheat pastry flour
- 1 cup (185 g) packed cooked white quinoa
- ¼ cup (48 g) chia seeds
- 1 teaspoon baking powder

- 1 teaspoon ground cinnamon Generous
- ¼ teaspoon fine sea salt
- Nonstick cooking spray

**Instructions**

- Before starting, here's a quick note: It's best to make sure that all ingredients are at room temperature when making the batter so that the coconut oil doesn't solidify when combined.
- Combine 1 cup (235 ml) of water and dates in a small saucepan. Bring to a boil, lower the heat, and cook on medium-high heat just until the dates start to fall apart; it should take about 2 to 3 minutes. Stir the coconut oil into the hot mixture to melt. Set aside to cool for at least 30 minutes. (Note that this can also be done in the microwave, using a deep, microwave-safe container and proceeding in 1-minute increments.)
- Add the remaining 120 ml of cup of water, maple syrup and vanilla and stir.
- Mix the flour, quinoa, chia seeds, baking powder, cinnamon and salt in a large bowl and stir to combine.
- Pour the wet ingredients over dry to mix. Let stand according to the manufacturer's instructions while heating the waffle maker.
- Waffle the iron easily with oil spray. 135 Add the waffle cup 135 cups (135 g) to two squares of waffle maker or follow the

manufacturer's instructions enough to cover the dough so that it does not overflow and that the waffles are well cooked.

- Close the waffle iron and bake for about 8 minutes until golden brown. Remove waffles from the iron and let stand on a cooling rack for at least 5 minutes until the waffles are crispy. Do not miss this step!

- Leftovers are even better: you can toast them in a toaster or toaster so that the waffles are crispy again. You can also freeze waffles for up to 3 months, until you squeeze them. Still freeze directly in the refrigerator or frozen toaster so they are hot and crispy.

# Salmon Stuffed with Lime, Cilantro, Anaheim Peppers, and Scallions

## Ingredients

- 1 whole salmon, cleaned and gutted, about 6 pounds (2.7 kg)
- 1 lime, sliced paper-thin
- 1 bunch cilantro, chopped
- 1 Anaheim chili pepper, cut in matchstick strips
- 3 scallions, sliced thin lengthwise

- 2 tablespoons (30 g) olive oil

**Instructions**

- Is simple. Heat the oven to 350 degrees Fahrenheit (180 degrees Celsius or gas 4). Put the salmon in a large saucepan sprinkled with non-stick cooking spray. Now pour everything except oil into salmon and distribute it evenly throughout the body cavity.

- I want to use salmon

- Hard needle and cooking cord. Rub it now with olive oil on both sides and bake 30 - 40 minutes. It is a good idea to stick a thermometer on the thick side of the meat to see if it is finished. It should read between 135 degrees Fahrenheit and 140 degrees Fahrenheit.

- Slice slices with a few slices of spices per serving.

**Yield:**

12 servings

Each with 45 grams of protein; 1 gram of carbohydrates; dietary fiber following 1 gram of carbohydrates.

## Turkey-Parmesan Stuffed Mushrooms

**Ingredients**

- 1-pound (445 g) SKI

- 2 und turkey ¼ cup grated (75 g) Parmesan cheese
- ½ cup (115 g) mayonnaise 1 teaspoon dried oregano
- 1 teaspoon dried basil
- 2 cloves garlic, crushed
- 1 teaspoon salt or Vege-Sal
- ¼ teaspoon pepper
- 1½ pounds (670 g) mushrooms

**Instructions**

- Heat the oven to 350 degrees F (180 degrees Celsius or gas 4).
- Mix turkey, parmesan, mayonnaise, oregano, basil, garlic, salt and pepper and mix well.
- Clean the mushrooms with a damp cloth and remove the stems.
- Pour the mixture into the mushroom doors and place in a shallow bowl. Add just enough water to cover the pot, cook for 20 minutes and serve hot.
- Yield: About 45 mushrooms
- Each contains 1 gram of carbohydrates, one trace of fiber and 3 grams of protein.

# Saffron "Rice"

## Ingredients

- ½ head cauliflower
- 1 teaspoon saffron threads
- ¼ cup (60 ml) water
- ½ medium onion, chopped
- 1 teaspoon minced garlic or 2 cloves garlic, crushed
- 2 tablespoons (28 g) butter
- 2 teaspoons chicken bouillon granules
- ¼ cup (30 g) chopped toasted almonds

## Instructions

- Run the cauliflower using a food processor with a razor blade. Put the cauliflower in a microwave oven, add a few tablespoons (30 ml) of water, and cover the microwave for 7 minutes over high heat.
- Start soaking the saffron wires in the water. While this is happening, pour the onion and garlic in medium heat butter into a large, heavy fish.

- When the cauliflower is over, remove it from the microwave, drain it and add it to the fish. Pour in water and saffron and mix in the chicken seeds. Allow it to cook for a minute or two as you crush the almonds. Pour almonds into the rice and serve.

**Yield:**

5 servings of bright "rice" yellow

Each with 4 grams of carbohydrates and 1 gram of fiber, for a total of 3 grams of usable carbohydrates and 2 grams of protein.

Sides

# Cauliflower Puree

### Ingredients

- 1 head cauliflower or 1/8 pounds (680 g) frozen cauliflower
- 4 tablespoons (56 g) butter
- Salt and pepper

### Instructions

- Cover the jar with a lid, a few tablespoons (30 ml) of water and cover. Boil it for 10 to 12 minutes or until chilled, but it doesn't smell. (You may want to steam or cook the cauliflower if you wish.) Empty it completely and place it in a mixer or pan to cook well. Add butter, salt and pepper to taste.

- Yield: At least 6 generous portions
- Each contains 5 grams of carbohydrates and 2 grams of fiber, for a total of 3 grams of usable carbohydrates and 2 grams of protein.

## Chipotle-Cheese Fauxtatoes

### Ingredients

- 1 large chipotle Chile canned in adobo, minced; reserve 1 teaspoon sauce
- ½ cup (60 g) shredded Monterey Jack cheese
- 1 batch The Ultimate Fauxtatoes

### Instructions

- Slice a teaspoon of Edobo sauce and place the chopped cheese in the final pepperoni bread. Serve immediately!
- Each with 14 grams of protein; 14 grams of carbohydrates; 8 grams of dietary fiber; 6 grams of carbohydrates.

## Cheddar-Barbecue Fauxtatoes

### Ingredients

- ½ head cauliflower, cut into florets

- ½ cup (120 ml) water
- ½ cup (55 g) shredded cheddar cheese
- 2 teaspoons Classic Barbecue
- Rub or purchased barbecue rub
- 2 tablespoons (10 g) Ketatoes mix

**Instructions**

- Insert cauliflower into your slow cooker, including stems. Cover the slow cooker, place it on a high surface and cook for 3 hours. (Or bake 5 to 6 hours.)
- When it's time, use a spoon to remove the cauliflower from the slow cooker and place it in the mixer or food processor (hold the S blade in place) and place it in the Nymph there or you can pull the water out and use a hand mixer to bite cauliflower right in the pot. Let the cauliflower drain and clean it!
- Mix everything to melt the cheese.

**Yield:**

3 servings

Each with 8 grams of protein, 6 grams of carbohydrates, 3 grams of dietary fiber, 3 grams of usable carbohydrates.

# Hobo Packet

## Ingrediants

- ½ head cauliflower
- ½ medium onion
- 1 medium carrot
- 1 large rib celery
- ½ teaspoon salt
- ½ teaspoon pepper
- 8 slices bacon, cooked
- 2 tablespoons (28 g) butter

## Instructions

- Start the fire on the coal or heat a gas stove.
- Chop the cauliflower into small pieces. Finely chop the onion, thicken the carrots one centimeter (6 mm) and chop the celery to a uniform thickness.
- Pour an 18 cm (45 cm) heavy aluminum foil onto the countertop. Collect vegetables in the middle. Sprinkle with salt and pepper, crush

- Bake the boiled bacon on top and fry it with butter. Bend the foil everywhere and sew several times to seal it well. Turn the end to close them.

- Pour the whole package on the grill and cook for about 12-15 minutes over medium heat or on the stove. Bend the package with a knife, place it on a plate to open and serve.

**Yield:**

6 servings

Each serving contains 3 grams of carbohydrates and 1 gram of fiber, 2 grams for usable carbohydrates. 3 grams of protein.

# Cauliflower Kugel

**Ingredients**

- 2 packages (10 ounces, or 280 g each) frozen cauliflower, thawed
- 1 medium onion, chopped
- 1 cup (225 g) cottage cheese
- 1 cup (120 g) shredded cheddar cheese
- 4 eggs
- ½ teaspoon salt or Vege-Sal
- ¼ teaspoon pepper Paprika

## Instructions

- Preheat oven to 350 °F (180 °C or gas mark 4).

- Chop cauliflower into pieces of ½ (1.3 cm). Mix in a large bowl with onion, muffins, cheddar, eggs, salt and pepper and mix well.

- Spray an 8-inch (20 20 20 cm) pan with nonstick cooking spray and spread the cauliflower mixture evenly downwards. Gently sprinkle the paprika on top and bake for 50 to 60 minutes or until the coagulant is set and light brown.

## Yield:

9 servings of 2 grams of fiber, 3 grams of usable carbohydrates and 10 grams of protein.

# Little Mama's Side Dish

This is just the thing with a simple dinner of broiled chops or a steak, and it's even good all by itself It's beautiful to look at, too, what with all those colors.

## Ingredients

- 4 slices bacon
- ½ head cauliflower
- ½ green pepper
- ½ medium onion

- ¼ cup (30 g) sliced stuffed olives

## Instructions

- It is fried in a large, heavy, medium-medium heat. (First, give the fisherman a jar of non-stick cooking spray.)

- Chop cauliflower into 1.3 cm V2 inch slices. Also, remove the stalk. Put the shredded cauliflower in a microwave-safe pot without lid, without wasting it, add a spoon (30 ml) of water, and cover the microwave for 7 minutes.

- Mix the bacon and then return to the plywood. Grease the peppers and onions. Already some fat is cooked from the bacon and begins to brown around the edges. Add the pepper and onion to the pan. Strain until the onion is translucent and the peppers begin to soften.

- The caution must be taken until the confluence of events ceases. Add it to the pot without stirring - mix a little extra water to dissolve the bacon aroma from the bottom of the pot and pour it into the pan with olive oil, leave it to cook for another minute. cook. When stirred, then serve.

**Yield:**

4 or 5 servings

Assuming 5 servings, each contains 3 grams of carbohydrates and 1 gram of fiber, for a total of 2 grams of usable carbohydrates and 2 grams of protein.

## Gratin of Cauliflower and Turnips

### Ingrediants

- 2 ½ cups (375 g) turnip slices
- 2 ½ cups (375 g) sliced cauliflower
- 1 ½ cups (360 ml) carb countdown dairy beverage
- ¼ cup (60 ml) heavy cream
- ¼ cup (90 g) blue cheese, crumbled
- ½ teaspoon pepper
- ½ teaspoon salt
- 1 teaspoon dried thyme Guar or xanthan (optional)
- ¼ cup (25 g) grated Parmesan cheese

### Instructions

- Preheat the oven to 375 degrees Fahrenheit (190 degrees Celsius or marked gas 5).
- Combine the shuttle and the cauliflower into a bowl to make sure they are almost evenly aligned.

- In a small saucepan over low heat, heat the dairy and heavy cream to warm up, add the blue cheese, pepper, salt and thyme. Stir until the cheese is melted. It is good to thicken this sauce with guar or xanthan.

- Spray a pot with non-stick cooking spray. Put about one third of cauliflower flowers and turnips in the pan and pour one third of the sauce evenly over them and make two layers of vegetables and sauce. Sprinkle parmesan on top. Bake for 30 minutes.

**Yield:**

6 servings

Each with 7 grams of protein; 8 grams of carbohydrates; 3 grams of dietary fiber; 5 grams of usable carbohydrates.

## Mushrooms in Sherry Cream

This is rich and flavorful and best served with a simple roast or the like.

**Ingredients**

- 8 ounces (225 g) small, very fresh mushrooms
- ¼ cup (60 ml) dry sherry ¼ teaspoon salt or Vege-Sal, divided
- ½ cup (115 g) sour cream 1 clove garlic 1/8 teaspoon pepper

**Instructions**

- Clean the mushrooms and remove the wooden ends from the stems.

- Put the mushrooms in a small saucepan with sherry and sprinkle with 1/8 teaspoon salt.

- Bring the pears to a boil, reduce the heat, cover the pan and allow the mushrooms to boil for only 3-4 minutes and shake the pan once or twice while cooking.

- In another small skillet over low heat, mix 1/8 teaspoon of salt, cream, garlic and pepper. You want to heat the cream through it, but don't let it boil or separate.

- When the mushrooms are finished, pour the liquid into a small bowl. After the cream has warmed, spoon it over the mushrooms and mix everything over medium heat. If it looks a little thick, add a teaspoon or two of the stored liquid.

- Stir in mushrooms and cream for 2 to 3 minutes over low heat, again making sure the cream does not boil or serve.

**Yield:**

3 servings

Each with 4 grams of carbohydrates and 1 gram of fiber, for a total of 3 grams of usable carbohydrates and 2 grams of protein

# Avocado Cream Portobellos

**Ingredients**

- 6 small portobello mushrooms
- ¼ cup (60 ml) olive oil 2 cloves garlic
- 1 tablespoon (4.2 g) dried thyme
- 2 dashes hot pepper sauce
- 1 small black avocado
- 3 tablespoons (45 g) sour cream
- 2 tablespoons (20 g) minced red onion
- Salt
- 6 slices bacon

**Instructions**

- Start the fire on the coal or heat a gas stove.
- Separate the stems from your portoblets (save them for cutting and serve for the tortilla or serve over the roast!) And place the mushroom covers on a plate. Measure the olive oil and chop one of the garlic cloves into it. Then mix the thyme and chili sauce. Using a brush, cover the launch caps on both sides with a mixture of olive oil.

- Next, cut the avocado, remove the pits and pour into a small mixer bowl. Fry it with a fork. Mix the cream, onion and other garlic cloves. Add salt to taste.

- Now we have to do your bacon cooking. Put it on a microwave bacon holder or on a glass plate and cook over high heat for 6 minutes (depending on your microwave power it may be slightly different).

- Grill the mushrooms while your bacon cooks! Place them on a slow charcoal oil stove or more than a medium and small gas stove. Roast for about 7 minutes or until the oil mixture is constantly beaten - you also want to use a bottle of water to put out the flames.

- When your mushrooms appear to be browning, place them back on your plate and extend them back into the kitchen. If it's not clear, give it another minute or two and then drain it. Divide the avocado mixture among the mushrooms, mixing it nicely and well. Chop and serve a slice of bacon on each stuffed mushroom.

**Return:**

6 servings

For every 9 grams of carbohydrates and 3 grams of fiber, there are 6 grams of usable carbohydrates. 6 grams of protein; 701

# Grilled Portobellos

**Ingredients**

- 4 large portobello mushrooms
- ½ green pepper
- ¼ small onion
- 1 clove garlic, crushed
- ¼ cup (60 ml) olive oil
- Salt and pepper
- ¼ cup (25 g) grated Parmesan cheese

**Instructions**

- Start a charcoal fire or preheat a gas grill.
- Separate the stems from your portoblet (save them to cut in the tortilla or drain to go on the stick) and place the lids on a plate.
- Cut both the green pepper and the onion and place in the food processor with the S blade. Add the garlic and pulse to coat everything relatively well. Add the olive oil and press again.
- Place the portobello on the side of the gill on a medium heat and brush with a little oil in the green pepper mixture - just put a brush in. Allow mushrooms to brown for 4-5 minutes. Turn them and

paste the green pepper and onion mixture into the pan for another 4-5 minutes. Watch out for the flaming olive oil! Sprinkle on a plate, sprinkle with salt and pepper and sprinkle each mushroom with 1 teaspoon (6.3 g) of parmesan. Service.

**Yield:**

4 servings

There are 9 grams of carbohydrates and 2 grams of fiber per portion of 7 grams of usable carbohydrates. 6 grams of protein

# Kolokythia Krokettes

## Ingredients

- 3 medium zucchinis, grated
- 1 teaspoon salt or Vege-Sal
- 3 eggs
- 1 cup (150 g) crumbled feta
- 1 teaspoon dried oregano
- ½ medium onion, finely diced
- I ½ teaspoon pepper
- 3 tablespoons (15 g) soy powder or (32 g) rice protein powder
- Butter

## Instructions

- Mix the grated pumpkin with salt in a bowl and allow to stand for an hour or more. Remove and drain the liquid.
- Mix and combine egg, feta, oregano, onion, pepper and soy powder
- Good.
- Spray a heavy spoon of fish with thick cooking spray, add 1 teaspoon (14 g) of butter and melt over medium heat. Fry the pumpkin stick with a spoon and turn it once during cooking. Add more butter if needed and keep the croquettes warm. The trick to this is to allow them to completely brown or tend to disappear before trying to rotate them. If a few separate, do not sweat it. The pieces will still have an incredible taste.

## Yield:

6 servings

2 grams of fiber, 4 grams of usable carbohydrates and 8 grams of protein.

Improve the preparation time for the dish by rolling a pumpkin and onion through a food processor.

Salads

# Autumn Salad

## Ingredients

- 2 tablespoons (28 g) butter
- ½ cup (60 g) chopped walnuts
- 10 cups (200 g) loosely packed assorted greens (romaine, red leaf lettuce, and fresh spinach)
- ¼ sweet red onion, thinly sliced
- ¼ cup (60 ml) olive oil 2 teaspoons wine vinegar
- 2 teaspoons lemon juice
- ¼ teaspoon spicy brown or Dijon mustard
- 1/8 teaspoon salt
- 1/8 teaspoon pepper
- ½ ripe pear, chopped
- 1 ½ cup (40 g) crumbled blue cheese

## Instructions

- Melt the butter in a small heavy saucepan over medium heat. Add the walnuts and

- Allow to fry in butter and mix for 5 minutes.
- While the walnuts are roasting and make sure you keep them and do not burn them, wash and dry the vegetables and place them in an onion salad pan. First sprinkled with oil. Then combine the vinegar, lemon juice, mustard, salt and pepper and add to the salad bowl. Discard to cover everything well.
- Melt the salad with pears, warm walnuts and crushed blue cheese. Service.

**Yield:**

4 generous portions

And 6 grams of fiber, for a total of 7 grams of usable carbohydrates and 10 grams of protein

# Classic Spinach Salad

## Ingredients

- 4 cups (80 g) fresh spinach
- 1/8 large, sweet red onion, thinly sliced
- 3 tablespoons (45 ml) oil
- 2 tablespoons (30 ml) apple cider vinegar
- 2 teaspoons tomato paste
- 1½ teaspoons Splenda ¼ small onion, grated

- 1/8 teaspoon dry mustard Salt and pepper
- 2 slices bacon, cooked until crisp, and crumbled 1 hard-boiled egg, chopped

### Instructions

- Wash and dry the spinach very well. Tears the bigger leaves. Combine the onion in a salad bowl.
- In a separate bowl combine oil, vinegar, tomato paste, espresso, onion, mustard and salt and pepper to taste. Pour the mixture over the spinach, onion and pour.
- Chop the salad with bacon and eggs. Service.

### Yield:

- 2 generous portions
- 2 grams of fiber, 5 grams of usable carbohydrates and 2 grams of protein.

## Spinach-Strawberry Salad

### Ingredients

- 1 pound (455 g) bagged, prewashed baby spinach
- 1 batch Sweet Poppy Seed Vinaigrette
- 1 cup (170 g) sliced strawberries

- 3 tablespoons (25 g) slivered almonds, toasted
- ½ cup (60 g) crumbled feta cheese

## Instructions

Put the baby spinach in a large salad bowl. Pour dressing and pour well. It is served and served with strawberries, almonds and feta.

## Yield:

4 servings

Each with 8 grams of protein; 11 grams of carbohydrates; 5 grams of dietary fiber; 6 grams of carbohydrates.

# Summer Treat Spinach Salad

## Ingrediants

- 2 pounds (910 g) raw spinach
- 1 ripe black avocado ¼ cantaloupe
- ½ cup (15 g) alfalfa sprouts
- 2 scallions, sliced
- French vinaigrette

## Instructions

- Wash and dry the spinach very well. Tears the bigger leaves.
- Slice avocado in half, cut into crust and crust and cut into slices.

- Peel and crush the cantaloupe or use melons.
- Add avocado and cantaloupe to spinach with cabbage and lucerne. Throw in Winagart just before serving.

**Yield:**

6 servings

Each with 11 grams of carbohydrates and 5 grams of fiber, for a total of 6 grams of usable carbohydrates and 5 grams of protein.

# Dinner Salad Italiano

**Ingredients**

- 1 head romaine lettuce, washed, dried, and broken up
- 1 cup (70 g) sliced fresh mushrooms
- ½ cucumber, sliced
- ¼ sweet red onion, thinly sliced
- ½ pound (225 g) sliced salami, cut into strips
- ½ pound (225 g) sliced provolone, cut into strips Italian or vinaigrette dressing
- 2 ripe tomatoes, cut into wedges

**Instructions**

Make a large salad bowl of salad, mushrooms, cucumbers, onions, salami and prolones. Roast with Italian tomato sauce or finger, then add and serve the chopped tomatoes.

**Yield:**

3 servings

Each with 17 grams of carbohydrates and 6 grams of fiber, for a total of 11 grams of usable carbohydrates and 36 grams of protein

# Chef's Salad

**Ingredients**

- 10 cups (200 g) mmailie, iceberg, red leaf, or any other favorite lettuce
- ¼ pound (115 g) deli turkey breast
- ¼ pound (115 g) deli ham
- ¼ pound (115 g) deli roast beef
- ¼ pound (115 g) Swiss cheese
- 1 green pepper, cut into strips or rings
- ½ sweet red onion, cut into rings 4 hard-boiled eggs, halved or quartered
- 2 ripe tomatoes, cut vertically into 8 wedges each

- Salad dressing

**Instructions**

- Serve good salad beds on 4 plates.
- Slice turkey, ham, beef and Swiss cheese into strips. (However, getting a relatively thick meat and cheese is good for that.) Do all this artistically on salad beds and season with peppers, onions, eggs and tomatoes. Let each diner add their own clothes.

**Yield:**

4 servings

Each contains 13 grams of carbohydrates and 4 grams of fiber, for a total of 9 grams of usable carbohydrates and 37 grams of protein.

# Vietnamese Salad

**Ingredients**

- 4 cups (80 g) m lettuce, broken up
- 4 cups (80 g) torn butter lettuce
- 3 scallions, sliced, including the crisp part of the green shoot
- 1 ruby red grapefruit
- 1 tablespoon (1.5 g) Splenda
- 3 tablespoons (45 ml) fish sauce

- 3 tablespoons (45 ml) lime juice
- 1½ teaspoons chili garlic paste
- 2 tablespoons (15 g) chopped peanuts
- ½ cup (32 g) chopped cilantro ½ cup (12.8 g) chopped fresh mint

**Instructions**

- Wash and dry the salad, combine and then divide it into 4 salad plates.
- Chop the onion and spread on the salad.
- Half cut the grapefruit in half and use a sharp knife to slice it to break it apart. Divide portions of grapefruit into salads.
- Mix Splenda, fish sauce, lemon juice and red pepper paste. Pour equal amounts of dressing on each salad. Then chopped ground peanuts, chopped cantaloupe and pepper and serve.

**Yield:**

4 servings

Each with 4 grams of protein; 14 grams of carbohydrates; 4 grams of dietary fiber; 10 grams of usable carbohydrates.

# Cauliflower Avocado Salad

## Ingrediants

- 4 cups (600 g) cauliflower
- 1 black avocado, peeled and diced
- ½ green bell pepper, diced
- 8 kg la mat a olives, pitted and chopped
- 4 scallions, thinly sliced, including the crisp part of the green shoot Sun-Dried

## Instructions

- Cut the cauliflower into 1.3 cm (1/2 inch) slices. Put it in a microwave bowl, add 1 teaspoon (15 ml) of water and cover. Microwave oven for a long time for 7 minutes.
- When the cauliflower is ready, drain it and pour it into a mixing bowl and set aside. Everything else, including sun-dried tomatoes and basil and chopped eggplant. Serve warm on a bed of salad.

## Yield:

6 servings

Each with 3 grams of protein; 11 grams' carbohydrates; 4 grams of dietary fiber; 7 grams of usable carbohydrates.

# Sour Cream and Cuke Salad

### Ingredients

- 1 green pepper
- 2 cucumbers, scrubbed but not peeled
- ½ large, sweet red onion
- ½ head cauliflower
- 2 teaspoons salt or Vege-Sal
- 1 cup (230 g) sour cream
- 2 tablespoons (30 ml) vinegar (Apple cider vinegar is best, but wine vinegar will do.)
- 2 rounded teaspoons dried dill weed

### Instructions

- Mushrooms, cucumbers, onions and cauliflower as small as possible
- It can be. The cutting blade works well in the food processor and saves you time, but do it with a good, sharp knife.
- Brush the vegetables well with salt and refrigerate for an hour or two.
- In a separate bowl, mix the cream, vinegar and dill and mix well.

- Remove the vegetables from the refrigerator, remove any water that has accumulated on the bottom of the pan and mix the cream mixture.

**Yield:**

10 servings

1 gram of fiber, 3 grams of usable carbohydrate and 1 gram of protein.

# Crunchy Snow Pea Salad

**Ingredients**

- 2 cups (150 g) snow peas
- 4 slices bacon
- 1 ½ cup (50 g) roasted, salted cashews
- 1 cup (160 g) diced celery
- 1 cup (150 g) diced cauliflower
- ½ cup (120 ml) ranch salad dressing
- ½ cup (120 g) plain yogurt
- 1 teaspoon spicy brown mustard

**Instructions**

- First you want to close the end of the snow pea and pull the ropes hard. Cut them into 1.2 cm (1/2 inch) pieces. Put the pieces of snow peas in a microwave bowl, add a spoon (15 ml) or water and cover with a plastic plate or foil. Just microwave for 1 to 2 minutes, then remove and uncover to stop the preparation.

- Put the bacon on the microwave bacon

- Tooth or on a glass foot plate, microwave on high surface for 4 minutes or until crispy, then drain.

- While the bacon is cooking, chop it raw. Combine all vegetables, including snow peas, in a bowl.

- Combine the dressing on the farm, the yogurt and the mustard. Pour over vegetables. Chop in bacon, add jars and throw again. Cool before serving.

**Yield:**

4 to 5 servings

Assuming that 4 will each have 8 grams of carbohydrates and 2 grams of fiber, 6 grams for usable carbohydrates. 5 grams of protein.

# Parmesan Bean Salad

**Ingredients**

- 1 pound (455 g) bag frozen, crosscut green beans
- ½ cup (80 g) minced red onion
- ¼ cup (60 ml) extra-virgin olive oil

- 5 tablespoons (75 ml) cider vinegar
- ½ teaspoon salt or Vege-Sal
- ½ teaspoon paprika ¼ teaspoon dried ginger
- ¼ cup (75 g) grated Parmesan cheese

**Instructions**

Boil or microwave green beans until clear.

Allow the beans to cool slightly and then mix the onion, oil, vinegar, salt, pepper, ginger and parmesan. Cool well and serve.

**Yield:**

4 servings

Each has 12 grams of carbohydrates and 4 grams of fiber, for a total of 8 grams of carbohydrates and 9 grams of protein.

**Fish and Seafood**

# The Simplest Fish

## Ingrediants

- 1 fillet (about 6 ounces, or 170 g) mild white fish
- 1 tablespoon (14 g) butter
- 1 tablespoon (3.8 g) minced fresh parsley
- Wedge of lemon

## Instructions

Melt the butter in a heavy foil pan. Add the fish fillets and beat carefully for 5 minutes on each side or until the fish is matte and lightly lightening.

Transfer to a serving platter over chopped parsley and serve with a lemon wedge.

## Yield:

1 serving

Effect of carbohydrates, without fiber and 31 grams of protein.

# Ginger Mustard Fish

## Ingrediants

- 4 (6 ounces, or 175 g) fish fillets, such as tilapia, cod, or orange roughly
- 4 tablespoons (56 g) butter
- 2 teaspoons minced garlic or 4 cloves garlic, crushed
- 2 teaspoons grated ginger
- 2 teaspoons spicy brown or Dijon mustard
- 1 tablespoon (15 ml) water

## Instructions

- In a large, heavy skillet, start the fish in butter over medium heat. It should be 4-5 minutes on each side. Take the fish on a plate.
- Add garlic, ginger, mustard and more
- Pour the water into the pan and shake everything well. Repeat the fish inside, carefully rotating it once to make sure both sides are familiar with the sauce. Let it cook for another minute and then serve. Remove the fish sauce.

## Yield:

4 servings

Each contains 1 gram of carbohydrates, one trace of fiber and 31 grams of protein.

## Aioli Fish Bake

**Ingredients**

- 1 fillet (about 6 ounces, or 170 g) of mild, white fish
- 2 tablespoons (30 ml) Aioli
- 1 tablespoon (6.3 g) grated Parmesan cheese

**Instructions**

- Preheat the oven to 350°F (180°C, or gas mark 4).
- Spray a shallow baking pan (an ideal jelly roll) with a colorless cooking spray. Right on the baking tray, sprinkle a thick fillet with Aioli and sprinkle with a tablespoon of parmesan. Carefully rotate the fillet and spread Aioli and sprinkle the remaining parmesan. Bake for 20 minutes.

**Yield:**

1 serving

1 gram of carbohydrates, one trace of fiber and 32 grams of protein.

# Chinese Steamed Fish

## Ingredients

- 12 ounces (340 g) fish fillets
- 2 tablespoons (30 ml) dry sherry
- 1 tablespoon (15 ml) soy sauce
- 2 teaspoons grated ginger
- ½ teaspoon minced garlic or 1 clove garlic, crushed 1½ teaspoons toasted sesame oil 1 or 2 scallions, minced (optional)

## Instructions

- Wrap the fish fillets on a piece of heavy aluminum foil and rotate the edges of the foil to create a lip.
- Mix sherry oil, soy sauce, ginger, garlic and sesame oil.
- Close a shelf - a cake cooling rack works well - in a large container. Pour about one centimeter (6 mm) of water into the bottom of the tray and increase the heat. Put the foil with the fish on it. Carefully pour the sherry mixture over the fish. Cover the pan well.
- Cook for 5 to 7 minutes or until the fish is slightly crispy. If desired, serve with onion rolled like a pot.

**Yield:**

2 servings

Each contains 2 grams of carbohydrates, fiber and 31 grams of protein. Each serving has only 195 calories!

# Wine and Herb Tilapia Packets

**Ingredients**

- 1½ pounds (680 g) tilapia fillets, cut into 4 portions
- 4 tablespoons (56 g) butter, divided
- ½ cup (120 ml) dry white wine, divided
- ¼ cup (16 g) minced fresh herbs (chives, basil, oregano, thyme, or a combination of these), divided
- Salt

**Instructions**

- Preheat oven to 350 ° F (180 ° C or gas mark 4).
- For each sheet, pour a piece of aluminum foil about 45 cm (18 cm). Place a tab in the center of the foil square and gently twist the edges of the foil. 1 teaspoon (14 g) butter, 2 teaspoons (30 ml wine), 1 teaspoon (4 g) chopped herbs and just a little salt.
- Wrap the foil around the fish, rotate the edges in the middle and down so that the packaging cannot fall into the oven. Repeat all 4 portions.

- Put the packages right on the stove rack - without pan and bake for 35 minutes.

**Yield:**

4 servings

Each with 2 grams of carbohydrates and 1 gram of fiber, for a total of 1 gram of carbohydrates and 31 grams of protein

# Broiled Marinated Whiting

## Ingredients

- 6 whiting fillets
- ½ cup (120 ml) olive oil
- 3 tablespoons (45 ml) wine vinegar
- 1 tablespoon (15 ml) lemon juice
- 1 teaspoon Dijon mustard
- 1 clove garlic, crushed
- ½ teaspoon dried basil
- ¼ teaspoon salt
- ¼ teaspoon pepper
- mustard, garlic, basil, salt, and pepper and mix well.

## Instructions

- Put the fillets in a large plastic bag and pour into the oil mixture. In the refrigerator for a few hours and rotate the bag from time to time.

- Preheat the meat. Separate the marinated fish. Bend about 20 cm (20 cm) over the fire for 4-5 minutes on each side or cook on a stove.

- While the fish is cooking, pour the remaining marinade into a saucepan, boil briefly and then serve as a sauce.

**Yield:**

3 servings

Each has a little over 1 gram of carbohydrates, fiber and 34 grams of protein.

If you are in a hurry or do not have all the ingredients to prepare this dish, use the Winnie Garret dressing (180 ml) instead.

## Whiting with Mexican Flavors

**Ingredients**

- 4 whiting fillets
- 2 tablespoons (30 ml) lime juice, divided
- ¼ teaspoon chili powder
- 2 tablespoons (30 ml) oil

- 1 medium onion
- 2 tablespoons (30 ml) orange juice
- ½ teaspoon Splenda
- ¼ teaspoon ground cumin
- ¼ teaspoon dried oregano
- 1 tablespoon (15 ml) white wine vinegar
- ½ teaspoon hot pepper sauce Salt and pepper

**Instructions**

- Put the white fillets on a plate and sprinkle with 1 teaspoon (15 ml) lemon juice and return to the pallet. Peel the fillets without the red pepper powder.
- Heat the oil in a heavy skillet over medium heat. Add the white fillets. Bake for about 4 minutes on each side, turning carefully or until cooked through. Take out a plate and keep warm
- Add the onion to the pan and turn it over medium-high heat. Bake onions for a few minutes, until they begin to color. Mix lemon juice, orange juice, coriander, cumin, oregano, vinegar and hot pepper sauce. Cook them all for a minute or two. Season with salt and pepper. Pour onion over fish and serve.

**Yield:**

4 servings

Each with 5 grams of carbohydrates and 1 gram of fiber, for a total of 4 grams of carbohydrates and 17 grams of protein

Each serving has only 162 calories!

# Brined, Jerked Red Snapper

**Ingredients**

2 pounds (910 g) red snapper fillets

**FOR THE BRINE:**

- 1 ½ cup (100 g) kosher salt
- 3 quarts (2.8 L) water
- 2 tablespoons Jerk Seasoning
- FOR THE SEASONINGS:
- 4 cloves garlic, crushed
- 8 teaspoons olive oil
- 1 rounded tablespoon Jerk Seasoning
- ¼ cup (60 ml) lemon juice
- 4 teaspoons soy sauce
- 4 scallions, sliced

**Instructions**

- To make brine: In a deep, inactive container large enough to hold fish fillets, dissolve the salt in water - it becomes easier if the water is heated in a hot sauce. If you have used hot water, allow it to be no hotter than hot water before adding fish fillets. Make sure they are submerged in the brine and allow them to stand in the fridge for 1-2 hours.

- Well, the time is up. Start the fire on the coal or heat a gas stove. Drain the brine from your fish. In a small plate or pie, mix the garlic and olive oil, then mix in the chopped peppers, lemon juice and soy sauce. Reserve a little marinade, place the rice fillets over the remaining marinade and turn them once or twice. Allow the fillets to stand for 15 minutes or longer. Then fry over medium heat, 3-5 minutes on each side. When spinning the fish, reserve both sides with a spice mixture.

- When the fish is out, remove the serving plates and sprinkle each fillet with a chopped onion

**Yield:**

4 servings

For each serving of 4 grams of carbohydrates and 1 gram of fiber, 3 grams of usable carbohydrates (if you use a sour spicy recipe). 41 grams of protein

# Lemon-Mustard Salmon Steaks

## Ingredients

- 2 salmon steaks (totaling about 1 pound, or 455 g)
- 2 tablespoons (28 g) butter
- 1 tablespoon (15 ml) lemon juice
- 1 teaspoon Dijon mustard
- 1 pinch salt or Vege-Sal
- 2 tablespoons (7.8 g) chopped fresh parsley

## Instructions

- Combine butter, lemon juice, mustard and salt or Vege-Salt in a slow cooker. Cover the slow cooker, lower it and cook for 30 to 40 minutes. Mix with.
- Now place the salmon steaks in the slow cooker and wrap them once or twice. Cover the slow cooker again and cook for 1 hour. Peel the potato juice over the salmon and sprinkle the parsley before serving.

## Yield:

2 servings

Each contains 46 grams of protein, 1 gram of carbohydrate, dietary fiber tracking, 1 gram of carbohydrate.

# Curried Shrimp in Coconut Milk

## Ingredients

- 1 pound (455 g) large shrimp, shelled (31/35 count)
- 14 ounces (425 ml) coconut milk
- 1½ tablespoons (9 g) curry powder
- 1 clove garlic, crushed
- 1 teaspoon chili garlic paste
- 1 tablespoon (15 ml) fish sauce
- 2 teaspoons Splenda
- 3 scallions, sliced thin
- ¼ cup (16 g) chopped cilantro

## Instructions

- In a large shallow saucepan, mix the coconut milk, curry powder, garlic and garlic paste with pepper. Heat over medium-high heat and leave on low heat for 7-10 minutes.
- Add shrimp, fish sauce and splendor. Stir another 5 to 7 minutes and kiss until the shrimp are completely pink.

- Stir the onion, let it boil for another minute and, if desired, add or similar to a tablespoon of cauliflower rice. Melt each portion with crushed cilantro.

**Yield:**

3 servings

Each with 29 grams of protein; 12 grams of carbohydrates; 4 grams of dietary fiber; 8 grams of carbohydrates.

Poultry and Beef

# Drunken Chicken Wings

## Ingredients

- 20 whole chicken wings, or 40 drummettes
- 1 tablespoon (15 ml) fish sauce
- 1 tablespoon (6 g) grated ginger
- 2 teaspoons black pepper
- 1 teaspoon chili garlic paste ¼ cup (6 g) Splenda
- 2 tablespoons (30 ml) sugar-free imitation honey
- ¼ cup (60 ml) bourbon

## Instructions

- Dispose of the wings in a large plastic bag that can be used. Mix everything together. Reserve a marinade to lose weight and pour the rest on the wings. Press the air, seal the bag and throw it in the refrigerator. Allow the wings to survive for at least a few hours.

- When it comes to cooking, turn on the oven; When the fire is ready, pour the marinade and place the wings on the stove. Roast for 7-10 minutes on each side, often cooling with reserved marinade. Make sure to use clean utensils every time you use clean containers to prevent cross contamination.

- Service.

- Yield: You will definitely have 20 wings or 40 drums. It depends on whether you serve them as the main or the main.

- Each upper wing will have less than 1 gram of carbohydrates and 9 grams of protein. Half of these figures for drums. The carbon number does not include polyols in sugar-free honey.

## Greek Roasted Chicken

### Ingredients

- 3 to 4 pounds (1.4 to 1.8 kg) of chicken
- ¼ cup (60 ml) lemon juice
- ½ cup (120 ml) olive oil
- ½ teaspoon salt
- ¼ teaspoon pepper

### Instructions

- Wash the chicken and dry it with paper towels.
- Combine lemon juice, olive oil, salt and pepper and mix well. If using whole chicken, rub it with some of this mixture and make

sure you rub it in the body cavity a lot. If using chopped chicken, place it in a large plastic bag, pour the marinade over it and seal the bag.

- Leave the chicken to marinate for at least one hour or until the day.

- Remove the chicken from the bag at least 1 hour before serving. You can grill your chicken or bake it at 375 degrees Fahrenheit (190 degrees Celsius, or 5 marks) for about 1 hour. Anyway, cook it so that the fruit juices are not pierced when they are pierced into the bone.

**Yield:**

5 servings

Each with less than 1 gram of carbohydrates, one trace of fiber and 52 grams of protein

# Korean Barbecued Chicken

**Ingredients**

- 2 pounds (910 g) chicken pieces
- 2 tablespoons (33 g) chili garlic paste
- 3 tablespoons (45 ml) dry sherry
- 1 tablespoon (15 ml) soy sauce

- 4 cloves garlic, crushed
- 1½ tablespoons (23 ml) toasted sesame oil
- 1 tablespoon (6 g) grated ginger
- 2 scallions, minced
- 2 teaspoons black pepper
- 1 tablespoon (1.5 g) Splenda plastic bag.

**Instructions**

- Mix everything together. Reserve a little marinade to be weak and pour the rest over the chicken. Press the air, seal the bag and throw it in the refrigerator. Allow the chicken to marinate for a few hours.

- When it's time to cook, heat the oven. You want it in the medium to medium range. When the oven is ready to cook, remove the chicken from the bag and pour the marinade. Cook on the chicken side for 12 to 15 minutes and keep the grill closed, except for bending. Turn it on the skin and allow it to cook 7 - 9 minutes, again, with the grill closed. Turn it on the skin and leave it on the grill, so that the water does not turn on when it is bone and pierces it.

- The thermometer reads 180 degrees Fahrenheit (85 degrees Celsius) with instant reading. The reserved marinated dish several times during cooking, make sure you use clean dishes every time you eat. Drizzle the remaining marinade and serve the chicken.

**Yield:**

4 servings

With all the marinade, each serving contains 4 grams of carbohydrates and 1 gram of fiber, but you will not eat the whole marinade. No more than 3 grams per serving. 30 grams of protein.

# Cinnachick

## Ingredients

- 1 broiler-fryer, cut up—about 2 ½ to 3 pounds (1.1 to 1.4 kg)
- ½ cup (120 ml) dry sherry
- 3 tablespoons (45 ml) sugar-free imitation honey
- 3 tablespoons (4.5 g) Splenda
- 2 teaspoons ground cinnamon 1 teaspoon curry powder
- 1 clove garlic, crushed ½ teaspoon salt

## Instructions

- Simply mix everything except the chicken and put a little marinade to taste and pour the remaining chicken in a shallow pan, inactive or in a plastic bag. If using a bag, squeeze the air and seal it. Put the chicken in the fridge and let it marinate anywhere from a few hours to a full day.

- Then heat an average grill for a fine-grained gas or coal grill in a heavy-charcoal grill. Cool the chicken bone for 12 minutes, then rotate it for 7 or 8 minutes. Keep the bonnet closed, unless you rotate the chicken or avoid extinguishing the flames with the squirrel vial. Rotate it again and grill to clean the chicken water while drilling. Each time you eat, reserve the chicken with the marinade and drain into a clean container.

**Yield:**

4 servings

Each has 4 grams of carbohydrates and does not use many drops in honey imitation. 1 gram of fiber. However, these figures mean that you will consume all the marinades that you will not win, so I would not guess more than 2 grams per serving; 36 grams of protein

# Tarragon Chicken

## Ingredients

- 1 cut up broiler-fryer
- 2 tablespoons (28 g) butter
- 1 teaspoon salt or Vege-Sal Pepper
- 3 tablespoons (4.8 g) dried tarragon leaves

- 1 clove garlic, crushed
- ½ cup (120 ml) dry white wine

**Instructions**

- If your baby is in a quadrant, cut off the legs from the thighs and the wings from the breasts. (This method easily matches your skill set.)
- Melt the butter in a heavy skillet over medium heat and roast the chicken and turn it once or twice until golden.
- Pour more fat and sprinkle with salt and just a slice of water
- Slice the tarragon pepper over the chicken and gently crush it between your fingers to release the taste, then add the garlic and wine.
- Cover the bottom of the pan, reduce the heat and boil for 30 minutes and rotate the chicken at least once. When serving, pour a little pan on each piece of chicken.

**Yield:**

4 servings

Each contains 2 grams of carbohydrates, fiber and 44 grams of protein.

# Curried Chicken

## Ingredients

- 4 or 5 chicken quarters, cut up and skinned
- 1 medium onion
- 1 tablespoon (28 g) butter
- 1 rounded (6 g) tablespoon curry powder
- 1 cup (240 ml) heavy cream
- 3 or 4 cloves of garlic, crushed
- ½ cup (120 ml) water

## Instructions

- Heat the oven to 375 degrees Fahrenheit (190 degrees Celsius or gas mark 5).
- Arrange the chicken in a shallow pan and chop the onion and chop it over the chicken.
- Melt the butter in a small, heavy plate and pour the powder into it for a few minutes - just until it smells good.
- Mix the cream, garlic, water and curry powder over the chicken and cook for 1 hour to 1 hour and 20 minutes and turn the chicken every 20 to 30 minutes to cover both sides.

- To serve, place the chicken on a plate. Pour the sauce into the pan (it looks awful and kind of banana, but it will smell like heaven) and put it all in your mixer. If necessary, mix it with a little water or cream to get a nice, rich, golden sauce. Pour over the chicken and serve.

**Yield:**

4 generous portions

Each with 6 grams of carbohydrates and 1 gram of fiber, for a total of 5 grams of usable carbohydrates and 42 grams of protein

# Pizza Chicken

## Ingredients

- 3 chicken quarters, either legs or thighs
- 1 to 2 tablespoons (15 to 30 ml) olive oil
- 1 can (8 ounces, or 225 g) plain tomato sauce
- 1 can (4 ounces, or 115 g) mushrooms, drained
- ½ cup (120 ml) dry red wine
- 1 green pepper, chopped
- 1 small onion, chopped
- 1 or 2 cloves garlic, crushed, or 1 to 2 teaspoons jarred chopped garlic in oil

- 1 to 1/8 teaspoons dried oregano
- 3 ounces (85 g) shredded mozzarella cheese
- Parmesan cheese (optional)

**Instructions**

- Separate the chicken skin and cut the fourth leg and thigh in two parts into the leg joint.
- Heat the olive oil in a large heavy saucepan and heat the chicken over medium-high heat.
- Pour tomato sauce, mushrooms and wine. Add the green pepper, onion, garlic and oregano. Cover everything, turn the heat down and forget about 45 minutes to 1 hour.
- When the chicken is cooked, remove the fish from the fish and place on a serving platter. If the sauce is not good and thick, warm to medium and let the sauce boil for a few minutes.
- As the sauce thickens, sprinkle the chopped mozzarella and heat each plate for 20 to 30 seconds on the microwave oven with 50% power to melt the cheese. (Microwave oven may take a little longer or longer.)
- Pour the sauce over each slice of chicken and serve. If desired, sprinkle a little parmesan on the pizza chicken.

**Yield:**

3 servings

Each has 16 grams of carbohydrates and 4 grams of fiber, for a total of 12 grams of usable carbohydrates and 49 grams of protein.

# Chicken Tenders

## Ingredients

- 1 pound (455 g) boneless, skinless chicken breast
- 1 egg
- 1 tablespoon (15 ml) water
- ¼ cup (85 g) low-carb bake mix
- ½ teaspoon salt
- ¼ teaspoon pepper
- ½ cup (80 ml) oil

## Instructions

- Cut the chicken breasts about 1 cm (2.5 cm) long and 2 cm (5 cm) long. Beat the egg with water in a bowl. On a plate, combine baking powder with salt and pepper. Heat the oil in a heavy skillet over medium heat.

- Dip each piece of chicken in the egg wash, dissolve in the spice mixture and pour in the hot oil. Roast them until golden and serve with one of the sauces dipped in spices and spices.

# Chicken Sancocho

**Yield:**

4 servings

Each has 5 grams of carbohydrates and 2 grams of fiber, for a total of 3 grams of carbohydrates (excluding dipping sauces) and 40 grams of protein.

## Ingredients

- 1 whole chicken, about 5 to 5 ½ pounds (2.3 to 2.5 kg)

**FOR THE MARINADE:**

- 4 tablespoons (60 ml) lime juice
- 1½ cups (180 g) diced celery
- 1 large ripe tomato
- 1 medium onion
- 1 medium green pepper
- ½ tablespoon (2.3 g) poultry seasoning
- ½ teaspoon ground nutmeg
- 1 tablespoon ground cumin

**FOR THE STEW:**

- 1 quarter (960 ml) chicken liquid

- 1 large carrot, chopped
- 1½ cups (210 g) cube rutabaga
- 1½ cups (175 g) pumpkin cubes
- 1 small pot, cubes
- 1 cup (150 g) cauliflower and strain, cut into small pieces
- 3 cups (225 g) minced cabbage
- 1 teaspoon to 1 tablespoon chili or aromatic sauce - if you can make it use Scottish sauce from the Caribbean!

**Instructions**

- Remove the wipes from the poultry body and place the chicken in the soup pot.
- To make the marinade: Put all the ingredients for the marinade in a food with the S blade (you want to cut everything into large pieces and clean the onion and pepper and all) and press until suspended. Pour this mixture over the chickens and use clean hands to rub it, including in the body cavity. Wrap the whole pot in the fridge and let it sit overnight, if you think about it, turn the chicken once or twice in a row.
- To prepare the stew: The next day, remove the pot from the fridge with the chicken, place it on the stove and pour the broth over the chicken. Cover, put everything on medium heat, bring to

a boil, let it lightly and boil for one hour. Turn it off and let the pot sit on the stove and cool.

- When it cools, remove the chicken from the broth (large tongs are good for this), place it on a plate and set aside. Take extra fat from the juice and use the vegetables from the pickles sk I used a Chinese peel, but if you want, you can pour it through a sieve. Make sure you squeeze all the vegetables from the vegetables before returning them to the pot!

- Put the broth on the stove and set the heat on medium. Mix carrots, turnips, pumpkins and turnips and boil for half an hour. While cooking, separate the chicken skin and remove. Then remove the meat from the bones, discard the bones and cut the meat into bite-sized portions. About 20 minutes before serving, pour the chicken, cauliflower and cauliflower into the pot, warm

- Pepper sauce. Add water, if needed, to keep the broth above the meat and vegetables. Boil for 20 minutes and serve.

**Yield:**

8 servings

Each with 41 grams of protein; 13 grams of carbohydrates; 3 grams of dietary fiber; 10 grams of usable carbohydrates - but this figure is actually a big chunk, because you cut some vegetables. I call it 8 grams per serving. There is also a lot of beta-carotene and calcium.

# Spicy Peanut Chicken

## Ingredients

- 2 or 3 boneless, skinless chicken breasts
- 1 teaspoon ground cumin
- ½ teaspoon ground cinnamon
- 2 to 3 tablespoons (30 to 45 ml) olive or peanut oil for sautéing (I think peanut is better here.)
- ½ smallish onion, thinly sliced
- 1 can (141/2 ounces, 410 g) diced tomatoes, undrained
- 2 tablespoons (32 g) natural peanut butter
- 1 tablespoon (15 ml) lemon juice
- 2 cloves garlic, crushed Fresh jalapeno, cut in half and seeded

## Instructions

- On a plate or plate, mix the cumin and cinnamon and then sprinkle the chicken breast on both sides.
- Put the oil in a heavy saucepan over medium heat and add the chopped chicken and onion, add a little coffee on both sides.
- While this is happening, place all the liquid and half of the tomatoes in the tomatoes, in a blender or food mix with peanut

butter, lemon juice, garlic and jalapeño. (Wash your hands after touching that hot pepper or you'll be bad at the next touch of your eyes!) Mix or process to mix.

- Pour this relatively thick sauce over the chicken (which you transformed at least once, right?), Add the remaining tomatoes from the can, cover, cover, reduce heat and cook for 10 to 15 minutes or until cooked through. The chicken is cooked through it.

## Yield:

approximately 3 servings

Each with 14 grams of carbohydrates and 1 gram of fiber, for a total of 13 grams of usable carbohydrates and 26 grams of protein

**Appetizers and Snacks**

# Chinese Peanut Wings

## Ingredients

- ¼ cup (60 ml) soy sauce
- 3 tablespoons (4.5 g) Splenda
- 3 tablespoons (48 g) natural peanut butter
- 2 tablespoons (30 ml) dry sherry
- 1 tablespoon (15 ml) oil

- 1 tablespoon (15 ml) apple cider vinegar
- 2 teaspoons Chinese Five Spice powder
- ¼ teaspoon red pepper flakes (or more, if you want them hotter)
- 1 clove garlic, crushed
- 12 chicken wings or 24 drumettes

**Instructions**

- Preheat the oven to 325°F (170°C, or gas mark 3).
- Put the soy sauce, espresso, peanut butter, sherry, oil, vinegar, spice powder, peppercorns and garlic in a mixer or food processor and mix well.
- If you have whole wings of chickens and want to "drill" them, do it now. (This is preferably required.)
- Arrange the wings in a large bowl, pour the mixed sauce over them and then return them to the garment on each side. Let stand for at least half an hour (one hour is even better).
- Bake the wings for one hour and rotate every 20 minutes during baking.
- When the wings are finished, place them on a serving platter and return the sauce from the pot to the mixer or processor. Just flatten again for a moment to line up and serve with wings.

**Yield:**

24 pcs

Each contains 1 gram of carbohydrates, one trace of fiber and 5 grams of protein.

# Southwestern Stuffed Eggs

## Ingredients

- 6 hard-boiled eggs
- 2 tablespoons (28 g) mayonnaise
- 1 tablespoon (15 g) plain yogurt
- 1 tablespoon (10 g) minced onion
- ¼ teaspoon chili powder
- 1 tablespoon (15 ml) cider vinegar
- IA teaspoon garlic, finely minced

## Instructions

- Peel the eggs and chop the eggs in half. Carefully mix the yolks into a bowl and place the egg whites on a plate.
- Chop the yolks well with a fork and then brown with mayonnaise and yogurt. When the mixture is even, mix other ingredients.
- Drag the mixture back to the egg whites. You can sprinkle some peppercorns or peppers to make them look beautiful.

**Yield:**

12 pieces

Each with 3 grams of protein; 1 gram of carbohydrates; dietary fiber following 1 gram of usable carbon.

## Chili Lime Wings

### Ingredients

- 1 tablespoon (7 g) paprika
- 1 teaspoon chili powder
- 1 teaspoon dried oregano, crumbled
- ¼ teaspoon salt
- ¼ teaspoon pepper
- ½ teaspoon garlic powder
- 1½ pounds (680 g) chicken wings
- 3 tablespoons (45 ml) olive oil 1 lime, cut in wedges

### Instructions

- Preheat oven to 375°F (190°C, or gas mark 5).
- In a small bowl, combine the pepper and the following 5 ingredients (with garlic powder).

- If you like "individual drums", cut your wings (or you can buy them). Arrange them in a bowl and oil them with olive oil. Now sprinkle the paprika mixture evenly on the wings.

- Roast at least 45 minutes and not be damaged for one hour. You want them crunchy! If you have cart wheels, this is a great way to cook these ingredients.

- Warm with lime wedges to press the wings.

**Yield:**

approximately 14 pieces

Each with 5 grams of protein; 1 gram of carbohydrates; dietary fiber tracking 1 gram of usable carbon.

# Fish Eggs

## Ingredients

- 6 hard-boiled eggs
- 2 tablespoons (28 g) mayonnaise
- 2 tablespoons (30 g) sour cream
- ¼ cup (50 g) moist smoked salmon, mashed fine
- 1 tablespoon (15 g) jarred, grated horseradish
- 2 teaspoons finely minced sweet red onion

- 1/8 teaspoon salt

**Instructions**

- Peel the eggs and chop the eggs in half.
- Carefully mix the yolks into a bowl and place the egg whites on a plate.
- Chop the yolks with a fork. In mayonnaise, mix cream, salmon, horseradish, onion and salt and mix until creamy. Drag the mixture back to the egg whites.
- Yield: 12 halves
- Each has a trace of carbohydrates, a trace of fiber and 3 grams of protein.

## Curried Chicken Dip

**Ingredients**

- 1 can (5 ounces, or 140 g) chunk chicken, drained
- 3 ounces (85 g) light cream cheese
- 1 tablespoon (14 g) mayonnaise
- 2 tablespoons (20 g) minced red onion
- ½ teaspoon curry powder
- 1 teaspoon brown mustard

- ¼ teaspoon hot pepper sauce, or to taste
- 2 tablespoons (10 g) minced fresh parsley

**Instructions**

Assemble everything in your food processor with the S blade in place and pulse to smooth. Put the impregnation in a beautiful bowl and surround it with cucumbers, celery sticks and / or strips of pepper.

**Yield:**

6 servings

Each with 7 grams of protein; 2 grams of carbohydrates; tracking dietary fiber 2 grams of carbohydrates. The carbon number does not include vegetable fats.

# Guacamole

**Ingredients**

- 4 ripe black avocados
- 2 tablespoons (20 g) minced sweet red onion
- 3 tablespoons (45 ml) lime juice
- 3 cloves garlic, crushed
- ¼ teaspoon hot pepper sauce
- Salt or Vege-Sal to taste

## Instructions

Half the avocado and pour the meat into a mixing bowl. Great with a fork.

Mix the onion, lemon juice, garlic, hot pepper sauce and salt to mix well to achieve the desired consistency.

## Yield:

6 generous portions

Each with 11 grams of carbohydrates and 3 grams of fiber, for a total of 8 grams of carbohydrates and 3 grams of protein

This recipe contains a lot of healthy fat and about three times more potassium in bananas.

# Dill Dip

## Ingredients

- 1 pint (460 g) sour cream ¼ small onion
- 1 heaping tablespoon (3 g) dry dill weed
- ½ teaspoon salt or Vege-Sal

## Instructions

Put the cream, onion, weeds and salt in a food processor to remove the onion. (If you do not have a food processor, chop the onion very well and mix everything together.)

You can serve this immediately, but if you let it cool for a few hours, it will taste even better.

**Yield:**

1 cup of 25 grams' carbohydrates and 1 gram of fiber, for a total of 24 grams of usable carbohydrates and 16 grams of protein per batch (this is easy enough for 10 to 12 people, so no one wants more than a few grams of carbohydrates.) And the analysis does not include vegetable fats.

# Worcestershire Nuts

**Ingredients**

- 1 cup (150 g) shelled walnuts
- 1 cup (100 g) shelled pecans
- 4 tablespoons (56 g) butter, melted
- 3 tablespoons (45 ml) Worcestershire sauce

**Instructions**

- Heat the oven to 300 degrees F (150 degrees Celsius or gas 2).
- Spread the nuts in a shallow pan and mix the butter, cover all the nuts.
- Roast for 15 minutes, then remove from the oven and mix the sauce.

- Roast for another 10 minutes.

**Yield:**

8 servings

Each 6 grams of carbohydrates and 2 grams of fiber, for a total of 4 grams of usable carbohydrates and 3 grams of protein.

# Smoked Almonds

## Ingredients

- 1-pound (455 g) almonds
- 3 tablespoons (42 g) butter
- 2 teaspoons Classic Barbecue
- 2 teaspoons salt 2 teaspoons liquid smoke

## Instructions

- Heat the oven to 300 degrees F (150 degrees Celsius or gas 2).
- Put a large, flat dish on a burner and melt the butter in it.
- Mix the spices, making sure they are mixed in butter.
- Now add the almonds and mix until well browned. Roast for 30 to 40 minutes. Store in reserved containers.

**Yield:**

12 servings

# Blue Cheese Dressing Walnuts

**Ingredients**

- 4 cups (400 g) walnuts
- ½ cup (120 ml) blue cheese salad dressing
- 1 teaspoon garlic salt

**Instructions**

- Combine the walnuts and dressing in your slow cooker. Stir until the walnuts are evenly coated with the sauce. Cover the slow cooker, lower it and boil for 3 hours, stirring once.
- Stir in the garlic before serving.

**Yield:**

16 servings

Each with 8 grams of protein, 4 grams of carbohydrates, 2 grams of dietary fiber, 2 grams of usable carbohydrates.

Desserts

# Bubble and Squeak

## Ingredients

- 1 tablespoon (14 g) butter
- 2 cups (150 g) shredded cabbage
- 1 medium carrot, shredded
- ¼ cup (120 g) chopped onion
- 1 batch The Ultimate Fauxtatoes
- ½ cup (60 g) shredded Cheddar cheese

## Instructions

- Preheat the oven to 350 degrees Fahrenheit (180 degrees Celsius or gas 4).

- Melt the butter in a large, heavy fish and smooth the vegetables until the onion begins to turn translucent and the cabbage becomes slightly soft.

- Spray a 6-liter (1.4-liter) plate with colorless cooking spray. Spread one third of the Fauxtato on the bottom, then make a half layer of the cabbage mixture. Repeat the layers and finish with a Fauxtato layer. Cheese top. Bake for 45 minutes and strain through all layers.

**Yield:**

6 servings

Each with 10 grams of protein; 14 grams of carbohydrates; 6 grams of dietary fiber; 8 grams of carbohydrates.

## Parmesan cheese

Run cauliflower through the food processor chopper. Put it in a microwave-safe bowl with a lid, add a few tablespoons (30 ml) of water, cover and simmer for 5 to 6 minutes. When you're done, discover it right away!

Combine olive oil and butter in a large, heavy-bottomed skillet over medium heat and mix until well combined. Add the mushrooms and smooth until the color is soft and changing. If the slices of mushrooms are large enough, you may want to break the edge of the spatula slightly when slicing.

When the mushrooms have softened, whisk and stir. Add eggs and brown rice and eggs - which will help with a little water to help mix the flavors. Mix well to distribute all the flavors.

Stir in the parmesan and serve.

**Yield:**

3 to 4 servings

Each will have 4 grams of protein. 2 grams of carbohydrates; 1 gram of dietary fiber; 1 gram of usable carbon.

# Thai Cucumber Salad

## Ingredients

- ½ small red onion
- 1 small, fresh jalapeno, seeds removed
- 3 medium cucumbers
- 2 or 3 cloves fresh garlic, crushed
- 2 tablespoons (12 g) grated fresh ginger
- ½ cup (120 ml) rice vinegar
- ½ teaspoon salt
- ¼ teaspoon pepper
- 2 tablespoons (3 g) Splenda

## Instructions

- Using a food processor with the S blade, place the onion and syrup solution in the food and press to crush both fine.
- Remove the S blade and place it on the cutting disc. Rotate the cucumbers and then pass them through the processor. (If you do not use a food processor, you want to fry the onion and run the jelly, then chop the cucumber evenly.)

- Put onions, pumpkins and cucumbers in a large bowl. In a separate bowl, combine the garlic, ginger, vinegar, salt, pepper and splendor. Pour the vegetables and mix well.
- Cool several hours before serving to get the best taste.

**Yield:**

8 generous portions

Each with 6 grams of carbohydrates and 1 gram of fiber, for a total of 5 grams of usable carbohydrates and 1 gram of protein.

# Mushroom "Risotto"

**Ingredients**

- ½ head cauliflower
- 3 tablespoons (42 g) butter
- 1 cup (70 g) sliced mushrooms
- ½ medium onion, diced
- 1 teaspoon minced garlic or 2 cloves garlic
- 2 tablespoons (30 ml) dry vermouth
- 1 tablespoon (6 g) chicken bouillon granules
- ¼ cup (75 g) grated Parmesan cheese
- Guar or xanthan

- 2 tablespoons (7.6 g) chopped fresh parsley

**Instructions**

- Run the cauliflower using a food processor with a razor blade. Put the cauliflower in a microwave oven, add a few tablespoons (30 ml) of water, and cover the microwave for 7 minutes over high heat.

- While the cauliflower cooks, it melts

- Put the butter in a large fish over medium heat and add the mushrooms, onion and garlic and mix together.

- When the cauliflower is ready, remove it from the microwave and drain it. When the mushrooms have changed and appear, add the cauliflower to the fish and mix everything. Mix in Vermouth, boil and cheese and cook for 2 to 3 minutes.

- Simply sprinkle some guar or xanthan on the "risotto", always mixing to give it a creamy texture. Stir in parsley and serve.

**Yield:**

5 servings

Each with 4 grams of carbohydrates and 1 gram of fiber, for a total of 3 grams of usable carbohydrates and 6 grams of protein

# Cauliflower-Olive Salad

## Ingredients

- ½ head cauliflower, broken into small florets
- ½ cup (80 g) diced red onion
- 1 can (2¼ ounces, or 60 g) sliced ripe olives, drained
- ½ cup (30 g) chopped fresh parsley
- ¼ cup (60 ml) lemon juice
- ¼ cup (60 ml) olive oil
- ¼ cup (60 g) mayonnaise
- ½ teaspoon salt or Vege-Sal
- About a dozen cherry tomatoes Lettuce (optional) and parsley in a bowl.

## Instructions

- Combine lemon juice, olive oil, mayonnaise and salt in a separate bowl. Pour the vegetables and pour well.
- It cools down for at least an hour - a whole day doesn't hurt. When the salad is ready, cut the cherry tomatoes in half and add them to the salad. Serve on a bed with salad, if you like, but it's great.

## Zucchini-Crusted Pizza

**Yield:**

4 servings

Each with 7 grams of carbohydrates and 2 grams of fiber, for a total of 5 grams of usable carbohydrates and 1 gram of protein.

### Ingredients

- 3 ½ cups (440 g) shredded zucchini
- 3 eggs
- 1 ½ cup (40 g) rice protein powder or (35 g) soy powder
- 1½ cups (175 g) shredded mozzarella, divided
- ½ cup (50 g) grated Parmesan cheese
- A pinch or two of dried basil
- ½ teaspoon salt
- ¼ teaspoon pepper Oil
- 1 cup (240 ml) sugar-free pizza sauce
- Toppings as desired (sausage, pepperoni, peppers, mushrooms, or whatever you like)

### Instructions

- Preheat oven to 350 ° F (180 ° C or gas mark 4).

- Sprinkle the pumpkin with a little salt and let stand 15-30 minutes. Put it in a straightener and press for extra moisture.
- Multiply the chopped pumpkin, eggs, protein powder, V2 cup (60 g) of mozzarella, parmesan, basil, salt and pepper.
- Spray a 9 13 13-inch (23 33 33 cm) pan with a non-stick cooking spray and spread the pumpkin mixture.
- Bake for about 25 minutes or until firm. Wash the pumpkin peel with a little oil and cook for 5 minutes until golden.
- Then spread the pizza sauce and add 1 cup (120 g) Mozzarella and other tops. (If you use vegetables as a topping, you may want to smooth them a bit at first.)
- Bake for another 25 minutes, then cut into squares and serve.

**Yield:**

4 generous portions

Each has 14 grams of carbohydrates and 2 grams of fiber, a total of 12 grams of usable carbohydrates and 22 grams of protein. (The analysis does not include toppings.)

# Broccoli Salad

### Ingredients

- ½ cup (120 ml) olive oil
- ¼ cup (60 ml) vinegar
- 1 clove garlic, crushed
- ½ teaspoon Italian seasoning herb blend
- ½ teaspoon salt or Vege-Sal
- ½ teaspoon pepper
- 4 cups (1 kg) frozen broccoli "cuts"

### Instructions

- Multiply the olive oil, vinegar, garlic, herbs, salt and pepper.
- They don't even bother you
- Broccoli - Put it in a bowl and pour the olive oil mixture over it. Stir well and let it sit in the refrigerator for a few hours. If you think and serve it as vegetables or vegetables, mix it.

### Yield:

6 servings

Each with 7 grams of carbohydrates and 4 grams of fiber, for a total of 3 grams of usable carbohydrates and 4 grams of protein.

Feel free to try fresh broccoli for this salad. You have to peel the stalks, cut and steam for about 5 minutes. And at that moment, it will melt just like frozen broccoli! I personally follow the easy way.

## Mixed Greens with Warm Brie Dressing

### Ingredients

- 6 cups (120 g) torn romaine lettuce, washed and dried
- 6 cups (120 g) torn red leaf lettuce, washed and dried
- 2 cups (40 g) torn radicchio, washed and dried
- 1 cup (60 g) chopped fresh parsley
- 4 scallions, thinly sliced, including the crisp part of the green shoot
- ½ cup (120 ml) extra-virgin olive oil
- ½ small onion, minced
- 3 cloves garlic, crushed
- 6 ounces (170 g) Brie, rind removed, cut into small chunks
- ¼ cup (60 ml) sherry vinegar
- 1 tablespoon (15 ml) lemon juice
- 1½ teaspoons Dijon mustard

### Instructions

- Put the salad, root, parsley and onion in a large salad bowl and refrigerate.

- Put the olive oil in a heavy skillet over low heat. Add the onion and garlic and boil for 2 to 3 minutes.

- It melts in Brie, one piece at a time, whistling constantly with a whistle. (At first it seems very scary, but don't sweat.)

- When all the cheese has melted, sprinkle Dijon with sherry vinegar, lemon juice and mustard. Let it boil for a few minutes, stirring constantly, until the dressing is smooth and thick. Pour over salad and pot.

**Yield:**

6 servings

Each with 7 grams of carbohydrates and 3 fibers, for a total of 4 grams of usable carbohydrates and 8 grams of protein.

## Snow Pea Salad Wraps

**Ingredients**

- 2 cups (150 g) snow pea pods
- 4 medium celery stalks, diced fine
- ½ cup (80 g) minced red onion
- ½ cup (60 g) chopped peanuts

- ¼ cup (60 g) mayonnaise
- ¼ cup (60 g) plain nonfat yogurt
- 1 tablespoon (15 ml) lemon juice
- 1/8 teaspoon cayenne
- 8 slices bacon, cooked and drained
- 24 lettuce leaves

## Instructions

- Break the end of the snow pea and pull each string. Cut them into pieces / 1.3 cm. After cutting, measure them before cutting.
- Put slices of peas in a microwave for just 1 minute with a teaspoon of water, lid and microwave. Discover the bowl immediately!
- Mix the snow peas in a bowl and add the chopped celery, onion and hazelnuts. Mix mayonnaise, yogurt, lemon juice and cayenne. Discard the vegetables and discard. Cut the bacon and chop again.
- Arrange four salad leaves on each plate - I like Boston salad for that. Pour a pot of snow pea salad next to a tablespoon of salad. To eat, pour the snow pea mixture on a salad leaf, wrap and eat.

## Yield:

6 servings

Each with 8 grams of protein; 8 grams of carbohydrates; 3 grams of dietary fiber; 5 grams of usable carbohydrates.

## Not-Quite-Middle-Eastern Salad

**Ingredients**

- ½ head cauliflower
- 2/3 cup (70 g) sliced stuffed olives
- 7 scallions, sliced
- 2 cups (40 g) triple-washed fresh spinach, finely chopped
- 1 stalk celery, diced
- 1 small ripe tomato, finely diced
- 4 tablespoons (15.2 g) chopped parsley
- ¼ cup (60 ml) olive oil
- 1 teaspoon minced garlic or 2 cloves garlic, crushed
- 1 tablespoon (15 ml) red wine vinegar
- 2 tablespoons (28 g) mayonnaise
- Salt and pepper

**Instructions**

- Run cauliflower using a food processor knife, place in a microwave oven, add a few tablespoons (30 ml) of water, cover the pan and cook for only 5 minutes.

- While cooking, place the olives, onions, spinach, celery, tomatoes and parsley in a large salad bowl.

- When the cauliflower has come out of the microwave, pour it into a rectifier and run it for a moment or two in cold water to cool. (You can cool the cauliflower instead, but it will take a long time.) Drain the cauliflower well and sprinkle with other vegetables. Add oil, garlic, vinegar and mayonnaise and pot. Add salt and pepper to taste, bake and serve again.

**Yield:**

6 servings

Each with 5 grams of carbohydrates and 2 grams of fiber, for a total of 3 grams of usable carbohydrates and 1 gram of protein

Sauces and Seasonings

# Tarragon Mustard Sauce

## Ingredients

1/4 cup sour cream

1/4 cup Dijon mustard

1/4 cup half-and-half cream

½ - 1 teaspoon dried tarragon

## Instructions

In a bowl combine all the ingredients except the pepper.

Warm up / starve on low heat until dissolved.

Heated spoon, fish or steak.

Sprinkle with extra pepper and tarragon.

## Yield:

1 cup

# Walnut Sauce

## Ingredients

- 1 cup of milk
- 1 big slice of white bread, crusts removed

- 2 cups (200 gr) of walnuts kernels
- ½ clove of garlic
- 1 tablespoon of parmesan cheese
- 5 tablespoons of light extra virgin olive oil
- 10 leaves of marjoram
- Salt
- Lukewarm water

**Instructions**

- Put the bread in a bowl and cover with milk. When it is completely wet, drain it into your hands and press it.
- Put sliced bread in a mixer with nuts, garlic, magnesium leaves, parmesan cheese and 2 cups of salt. Mix for a few minutes until the walnuts are well and evenly crushed.
- Add 5 tablespoons of olive oil and warm water for a thick, creamy sauce.
- When it's time to season the pasta (any type of pasta: dry pasta, handmade pasta, ravioli or pansotti - of course) remember to pre-season the water in a sauce with 4-5 tablespoons of hot water on which the pasta is boiling water and is remembered. Always, always, to save on a cup of boiling water to add in the past, only if it stays dry after the seasoning.

**Yield:**

about 1-2 cups

# Orange Butter Sauce

## Ingredients

- 2 oranges
- 1/2 cup white wine
- 2 teaspoons minced shallots
- 1/2 pound (2 sticks) unsalted butter
- Salt and white pepper

## Instructions

- Make the syrup with orange peel, orange juice, wine and shells.
- Crush half of orange (about 2 teaspoons) and marinate two oranges (about 4.3 cups).
- Put water, steak, wine and mussels in a saucepan over medium-high heat.
- Cook until the syrup is almost gone.
- Gently toss in butter: over low heat, mix in a tablespoon of butter constantly and constantly.
- Add salt and pepper to taste.

## Yield:

about 1 cup

# Vinegar Baste

## Ingredients

- 1 cider vinegar 1/2 c hot water
- 2 tbsp brown sugar 1 tbsp vegetable oil
- 1 tsp black pepper
- 2 tsp red chili flakes
- 1 tsp paprika
- 2 tsp salt
- 1/2 tsp mustard powder
- 2 tsp Worcestershire sauce
- 1 tbsp maple syrup

## Instructions

- Put brown sugar and hot water in a non-active bowl and mix well to dissolve.
- Add all other ingredients and mix to combine.
- Apply freely on minced or pulled pork and mix. In the fridge for up to a week.

**Yield:**

about 1 cup

# 28 Different Introductory WW Day Plans For Beginners

If you are like many people, you groan at the thought of doing day plan for different meals. While you know it is something you need to do, it does not mean you like it! Meal prep takes time, but if you look at preparing say your vegetables just once for the whole week, then you will find it easier to eat healthy home-cooked meals each evening. Some foods, some vegetables are easy to prepare ahead of time and save well.

In this chapter, I have shared an introductory weight watcher's day plan for beginners you can follow to achieve your set goals.

## Day 1:

Total Smart Points: 21

- Breakfast: Individual Egg and Spinach Bowl (2 points)
- Lunch: Skinny Taco Lettuce Boats (3 points)
- Dinner: Roast Beef with Seared Pineapple and Side Salad (11 points)
- Snack: Southwestern Kale Chips (5 points)

## Day 2:

Total points: 22

- Breakfast: Slow Cooker Hot-Chocolate Steel-Cut Oatmeal (6 points)
- Lunch: Slow Cooker Fiesta Chicken Soup (4 points)
- Dinner: Stuffed Bell Peppers (7 points)
- Snack: Snack Pretzel Stack (5 points)

## Day 3.

Total points: 25

- Breakfast: Skinny Strawberry Banana Bread (4 points)
- Lunch: Grilled Chicken and Blueberry Salad (9 points)

- Dinner: Skinny Chicken Taquitos (5 points) with Skinny Mexican Rice (4 points)
- Snack: Oven-Baked Zucchini Chips (3 points)

## Day 4.

Total points: 21

- Breakfast: Breakfast Egg and Veggie Muffins (6 points)
- Lunch: Hearty Kale Salad (6 points)
- Dinner: Clean Eating Pizza Lasagna Rolls (7 points)
- Snack: Baked Apple Chips (2 point)

## Day 5.

Total points: 27

- Breakfast: Skinny Strawberry Yogurt (5 points)
- Lunch: Mediterranean Tuna Salad (6 points)
- Dinner: Turkey Meatloaf Cupcakes with Mashed Potatoes (10 points)
- Snack: Kale Slaw with Toasted Walnuts (6 points)

## Day 6.

Total points: 20

- Breakfast: Vanilla Quinoa and Roasted Blueberry Breakfast Bowl (8 points)

- Lunch: Zucchini Bell Pepper Pizza (3 points)
- Dinner: Slow Cooker Balsamic Chicken (4 points)
- Snack: Slow Cooker Skinny Applesauce (5 points)

**Day 7.**

Total points: 24

- Breakfast: Wake Me Up, Keep Me Going Smoothie (6 points)
- Lunch: Skinny Taco Salad in a Jar (6 points)
- Dinner: Pasta Puttanesca with Baby Spinach (9 points)
- Snack: Baked Onion Rings (3 points)

**Day 8.**

Total points: 24

- Breakfast: Skinny Protein Breakfast Frittata (2 points)
- Lunch: Clean Eating Chicken Salad (6 points)
- Dinner: Lemon Chicken Breasts with Asparagus and Salad (11 points)
- Snack: Refreshing Lemon-Lime Popsicles (5 points)

**Day 9.**

Total points: 21

- Breakfast: Skinny Berry Parfait (11 points)

- Lunch: Pasta Salad with Pesto, Mozzarella and Tomatoes (4 points)
- Dinner: German Schnitzel, Slow Cooker Style (5 points)
- Snack: Paleo Friendly Meaty Veggie Roll Ups (1 point)

**Day 10.**

Total points: 23

- Breakfast: Overnight French Toast Casserole (8 points)
- Lunch: Supermodel Superfood Salad (6 points)
- Dinner: Asian Salad with Crispy Chicken (5 points)
- Snack: Skinny Bell Pepper Nacho Boats (4 points)

**Day 11.**

Total points: 28

- Breakfast: Banana-Walnut Bran Muffins (10 points)
- Lunch: Chicken and Crisp Veggie Sandwich (8 points)
- Dinner: Blackened Sockeye Salmon (5 points)
- Snack: Almond Butter and Banana Sandwiches (5 points)

**Day 12.**

Total points: 25

- Breakfast: Fried Eggs with Mushrooms and Brussel Sprouts (4 points)
- Lunch: Clean Eating Nut Butter and Jam Sandwich (5 points)
- Dinner: Mediterranean Penne with Sundried Tomatoes (9 points)
- Snack: Cranberry Pumpkin Seed Granola (7 points)

## Day 13.

Total points: 26

- Breakfast: Slow Cooker Sweet Potato Oatmeal (6 points)
- Lunch: Chickpea and Tomato Salad with Grilled Chicken (8 points)
- Dinner: Slow Cooker Herb Chicken and Vegetables (5 points)
- Snack: Chocolate Peanut Butter Protein Smoothie (7 points)

## Day 14.

Total points: 26

- Breakfast: Crustless Spinach Quiche with Sundried Tomatoes (4 points)
- Lunch: Mushroom and Steak Fajita Sandwiches (6 points)
- Dinner: Caribbean Mango Chicken Burgers (10 points)
- Snack: Quinoa Crisp & Berry Parfait (6 points)

**Day 15.**

Total points: 26

- Breakfast: Protein Salmon and Eggs on Toast (6 points)
- Lunch: Chicken Florentine Casserole (7 points)
- Dinner: Skinny Banana Split Protein Smoothie (8 points)
- Snack: No-Bake Lemon Berry Cups (5 points)

**Day 16.**

Total points: 23

- Breakfast: Arm and Red Pepper Mini Frittatas (3 points)
- Lunch: Veggie & Pesto Sandwich (8 points)
- Dinner: Blackened Skirt Steak BLT Salad (8 points)
- Snack: Almond Joy Pizzert Babies (4 points)

**Day 17.**

Total points: 28

- Breakfast: Clean Eating Refrigerator Oatmeal (8 points)
- Lunch: Overstuffed Veggie Sandwich (12 points)
- Dinner: Asian Salad with Crispy Chicken (5 points)
- Snack: Peanut Butter Banana Cups (3 points)

## Day 18.

Total points: 24

- Breakfast: Southwestern Protein Breakfast Burrito (9 points)
- Lunch: Fiesta Chicken Soup (4 points)
- Dinner: Chicken Caesar Wrap (8 points)
- Snack: Clean eating Deviled Eggs (3 points)

## Day 19.

Total points: 21

- Breakfast: Sweet Potato Pancakes (4 points)
- Lunch: Jalapeno Tuna Lime Salad (7 points)
- Dinner: Slow Cooker Turkey Stew (4 points)
- Snack: Caramel Pumpkin Spice Popcorn (6 points)

## Day 20.

Total points: 28

- Breakfast: French Toast Casserole (9 points)
- Lunch: Tomato, Hummus, and Spinach Salad Sandwich (7 points)
- Dinner: Chicken Salad Sandwich with Bok Choy, Red Grapes and Walnuts (9 points)

- Snack: Peanut Butter Yogurt Honey Dip (3 points)

**Day 21.**

Total points: 20

- Breakfast: Crustless Asparagus Quiche (2 points)
- Lunch: Healthiest Greek Salad (8 points)
- Dinner: Zucchini Ribbon Salad with Pine Nuts and Parmesan Shavings (7 points)
- Snack: Classic Cucumber and Tomato Salad (3 points)

**Day 22.**

Total points: 25

- Breakfast: Old-Fashioned Pancakes (5 points)
- Lunch: Chickpea Cucumber Salad (5 points)
- Dinner: Cheesy Chicken Enchilada Bake (14 points)
- Snack: Spicy Pumpkin Hummus (1 point)

**Day 23.**

Total points: 27

- Breakfast: Slow cooker apple cinnamon oatmeal (7 points)
- Lunch: Skinny Taco Salad in a Jar (6 points)
- Dinner: Italian Bulgur Pilaf with Toasted Pine Nuts (9 points)

- Snack: 3 Ingredient Peanut Butter Cups (5 points)

**Day 24.**

Total points: 26

- Breakfast: Potato, Apple, and Gruyere Tart (7 points)
- Lunch: Crockpot Cauliflower Fried Rice (5 points)
- Dinner: Spinach Sauté with Pine Nuts and Golden Raisins (2 points) with Crockpot Low-fat Beef Stew (7 points)
- Snack: No-Bake Almond Cranberry Energy Balls (5 points)

**Day 25.**

Total points: 26

- Breakfast: Toast with Peaches, Cream Cheese, and Honey (5 points)
- Lunch: Chicken Chili (6 points)
- Dinner: Honey Dijon Glazed Salmon with a Hint of Lemon (6 points)
- Snack: No-Bake Almond Joy Cookies (9 points)

**Day 26.**

Total points: 25

- Breakfast: Three Seed Berry Parfait (6 points)

- Lunch: Snow Peas with Pecorino Cheese, Pine Nuts & Honey (7 points)
- Dinner: Slow Cooker Lentil & Veggie Stew (7 points)
- Snack: Sweet and Spicy Nuts (5 points)

## Day 27.

Total points: 28

- Breakfast: Superfoods Smoothie (5 points)
- Lunch: Skinny Black Bean Flautas (7 points)
- Dinner: Zucchini Lasagna (12 points)
- Snack: Chocolate Coconut Almond Balls (4 points)

## Day 28.

Total Points: 26

- Breakfast: No Crust Zucchini Quiche (4 points)
- Lunch: Crockpot Low-fat Beef Stew (7 points)
- Dinner: Lemon Chicken Breasts with Asparagus and Salad (11 points)
- Snack: Strawberry Sunrise Smoothie (4 points)

## Shopping Guide and Food List

### Fruits

- Avocado (1/8 medium avocado)
- Banana- ripe (1/2 medium)
- Banana- unripe/green (1 medium)
- Banana-sugar/lady finger (1 firm)
- Blueberries' (20 blueberries)
- Breadfruit (1/2 fruit)
- Cantaloupe/Rock melon (1/2 cup)
- Carambola/Star Fruit
- Coconut (1/2 cup)
- Cumquats/Kumquats (4 pieces)
- Dragon fruit (1 medium)
- Durian
- Grapes, all types Guava- ripe
- Honeydew melon (1/2 cup)
- Kiwi fruit (2 small)
- Lemons & Limes (including juice)
- Longan (5 longans)
- Mandarin & Clementine
- Oranges
- Passionfruit (1 whole)
- Pawpaw
- Pineapple (1 cup)
- Plantain
- Pomegranate (1/4 cup seeds)

- Prickly pear
- Rambutan (2 rambutans)
- Raspberries (10 berries)

**Cereals & Grains**

- Bran, Oats & Rice (2 tbsp.)
- Buckwheat groats (3/4 cup)
- Cereal, Gluten-free without honey/dried fruit (1 cup)
- Flakes of corn (1/2 cup)
- Flakes of corn, gluten-free (1 cup)
- Flakes of quinoa (1 cup, uncooked)
- Millet (1 cup cooked)
- Rhubarb
- Strawberries
- Tamarind (4 pieces)

- Noodles, rice stick & brown rice vermicelli (1 cup cooked)
- Noodles. soba (l/3 cup)
- Oats (1/2 cup)
- Oats, quick (1/4 cup dry)
- Pasta (1/2 cup cooked)
- Pasta. Gluten-free (1 cup cooked)
- Polenta (1 cup cooked)
- Puffed amaranth (1 /4 cup)
- Quinoa, all types (1 cup cooked) Rice, all types (1 cup cooked)

## Flour

- Almond meal (1/4 cup)
- Buckwheat flour (2/3 cup)
- Corn/maize flour/starch (2/3 cup)
- Gluten-free flour (2/3 cup)
- Millet flour (2/3 cup)
- Potato flour/starch (2/3 cup)
- Qumoa flour (2/3 cup)
- Rice flour (2/3 cup)
- Sorghum flour (2/3 cup)
- Tapioca flour/starch (2/3 cup)
- Teff flour (2/3 cup)
- Yam flour (2/3 cup)

## Nuts & Seeds

- Almonds, Brazil nuts, hazelnuts, pecans & walnuts (10 pieces)
- Chestnuts (20 boiled or 10 roasted)
- Flaxseeds/linseeds (I tbsp.)
- Macadamias (20 nuts)
- Mixed nuts (20 nuts)
- Peanuts (32 nuts)
- Peanuts (1 tbsp.)
- Seeds- chia, egusi. poppy, pumpkin sesame (2 tbsp.)
- Seeds- sunflower (2 tsp)

## Drinks

- Beer (1 can or 375ml)

- Drinking chocolate, cocoa, cacao but not carob (2 big tsp)
- Coconut water (1/2 cup or 100ml)
- Coffee- black & espresso (2 shots)
- Coffee- instant (2 tsp)
- Juice- cranberry & tomato (200ml)
- Juice- fresh orange (1/2 cup)
- Spirits- gin. vodka & whiskey (30ml)
- Strong Tea- green, peppermint & white (not dairy) (1 mug or 250ml)
- Weak Tea- black, chai & dandelion on water (1 mug or 250ml)
- Wine- red & white (1 glass or 150ml)

## Herbs & Spices

- All herbs 8. spices, fresh & dried except garlic, onion or chicory (usually 1 tsp. check Monash app)
- Salt & Pepper
- Spice mixes (no garlic or onion)
- Stock without garlic or onion

## Meat, Fish. Eggs, Tofu & Legumes

- Any unprocessed meat, fish or eggs (without high FODMAP ingredients like onion or garlic).

- Dahl- chana & urid (1/2 cup)
- Chickpeas, butter and garbanzo beans- canned & rinsed (1/4 cup)
- Lentils- canned & rinsed (1/2 cup)
- Lentils- red 8. green, boiled (1/4 cup)
- Lima & mung beans (1/4 cup)
- Quom (75 g)
- Tempeh (100 g)
- Tofu- firm not silken (2/3 cup)

**Vegetables**

- Alfalfa (1/2 cup)
- Artichoke hearts, canned (1/8 cup)
- Arugula/Rocket Asian & Collard greens
- Aubergine/Eggplant (1/2 cup)
- 8amboo shoots Beans, green (12 beans)
- Beansprouts Beetroot (2 slices)
- Bell peppers/Capsicum (1/2 cup)
- Broccoli heads or whole (1 cup)
- Broccoli, stalks or whole (1/2 cup)
- Brussels sprouts (2 sprouts)

- Cabbage (1 cup • not savoy)
- Carrots
- Celery (5 cm stalk)
- Cetenac (1/2 medium piece)
- Champignons, canned (1/2 cup)
- Chard/Silverbeet (1 cup)
- Chicory leaves (1/2 cup)
- Chicory/Endive/Witlof (4 leaves)
- Chili, red or green (11 cm long)
- Corn (1/2 cob max)
- Courgette/Zucchini (1/2 cup)
- Cucumber (1/2 cup)
- Edamame beans (1 cup)
- Endive (4 leaves)
- Fennel bulb or leaves (1/2 cup)
- Galangal
- Ginger
- Kale
- Leek leaves (1/2 cup)
- Lettuce and Endive- all types Mushrooms, oyster (1 cup)
- Okra (6 pods)
- Olives, green or black (15 small)
- Parsnips
- Pickles/Gherkins in vinegar (5 pieces)
- Potato- regular
- Potato- sweet potato (1/2 cup)
- Pumpkin/Squash- Kent/Japanese

- Pumpkin/Squash-butternut (1/2 cup)
- Radish
- Sauerkraut, white (1 tbsp.)
- Sauerkraut, red (1/2 cup)
- Scallion/Spring onion (green tops)
- Seaweed/nori (2 sheets)
- Snow peas/Mangetout (5 pods)
- Spaghetti squash (1 cup)
- Spinach. baby (1 cup)
- Sprouts (1/2 cup)
- Spinach -English
- Tomatoes- regular
- Tomatoes, cherry (4 cherries)
- Tomatoes. Roma (l small)
- Tomatoes, sundried (2 pieces)
- Turnip, Swede, Rutabagas (1 cup)
- Water chestnuts (1/2 cup)
- Yam (1 cup)

## Sauces & Condiments

- BBQ sauce (2 tbsp.)
- Capers (1 tbsp.)
- Chutney (1 tbsp.)
- Aubergine/Eggplant dip (2 tbsp.)
- Mayonnaise (2 tbsp.)
- Mint sauce 8(Jelly (1 tbsp.)
- Miso paste (2 sachets)
- Mustard (1 tbsp.)
- Pesto sauce (1/2 tbsp.)
- Shrimp Paste (2 tsp)

- Soy. fish & oyster sauce (2 tbsp.)
- Sweet & Sour Sauce (2 tbsp.)
- Tahini (1 tbsp.)
- Tamarind paste (1/2 tbsp.)
- Tomatoes, canned (1/2 cup)
- Tomato sauce (2 sachets or 13g)
- Tomato paste (2 tbsp.)
- Vanilla essence (1 tbsp.)
- Vinegar- apple cider, malt, red wine, rice wine (2 tbsp.)
- Vinegar- balsamic (1 tbsp.) Wasabi (1 tsp)
- Worcestershire sauce (2 tbsp.)

# Weight Watchers Top 15 Tips And Tricks

First, you need to know your habits. To find out about your eating habits, look where you feel like you're eating healthy foods. Write them in the notebook. Keep a list of what you eat for a few days. When you feel tired, upset, tired, stressed, depressed, or anxious, ask yourself if you want to eat. If you do, before meals, ask yourself if you are starving. If the answer is no, just drink a glass of water. Also, find out that when people eat foods that are not on your schedule, you do not like your food and do not deviate from it.

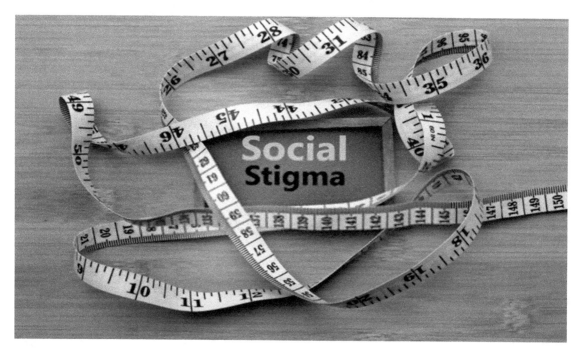

The next step is a gradual change. When you've identified the eating habits you want to change, remember that gradual changes work best.

When you realize that your eating habits are not as good as they should be, try to think positively. Changing eating habits can be enjoyable, and the health benefits will soon be evident.

I must say that the years I was and left weight Watchers have always worked for me! But it requires a lot of effort and commitment.

Here is my top 15 list for Observers' success.

**1. Keep a Diary** - This is a definitive piece! There is no way to pursue everything without one. You should update your newspaper with all the foods and drinks you consume daily. Most of the time, we tend to forget about the few snacks we had during the day. Always have a magazine handy, write it down with just a few sips or just a glass of wine.

**2. Liquids** - It is always a good idea to always have a bottle of water. This way you can eat all day on the water. And before you know it, you finally have 6 glasses of water to consume for 1 day. Sometimes, when you feel hungry, there is no need for food. You may only need water. So, if you want a snack, but this hunger doesn't fill you up, this is a wonderful thing. Water supply helps! And if the water does not do it for you, you have a slightly sweeter diet, and it can be much more than an old glass of water.

**3. Food / Snack** - Find several snacks and enjoy! They will help you when you feel your stomach is craving food. I like to have apples and carrots at work and home. Of course, you don't just have to eat these. But that's just what I like for a low or zero snacks. It's good to eat sweets and sweets now, but be sure you know how much chocolate candy they are.

**4. Food shopping** - Make a list! And before you go grocery shopping, before you go grocery shopping, make sure you know the amount of food you buy. It is a good idea to write down the value of the items you want to list next to each item on the list. If there is nothing on your list of where to find a supermarket, be sure to read its labels and sizes. Calculate those points!

**5. Cooking** - I like to stay healthier when cooking. For example, using "I can't believe" instead of ordinary butter is not butter. Use weak tools like weak chicken liquid. If you have salads, there are several types of fat-free fats. Just be smart!

**6. Weight and weight measurement** - **purchase scale**! I recommend the weight scale. Weigh in grams and ounces. Of course, you can use other scales, and I prefer just to use the weight scale. Seeing a 4 ounce is very shocking. Look at the sticky patch on the screen and see how small it is.

**7. Eating foods - make healthy choices**. If you enjoy your favorite food, which is +20 points, you should apply for food as soon as you prepare your meal. Put half of it in the pan and store it for lunch tomorrow. And if you need to make that piece of cheesecake for dessert, why not share it with your friend, instead of eating the whole slice yourself! And remember to follow my restaurant guide for points and points plus values.

**8- Friends and family** - Make sure they accompany you along the way to help you with your weight loss journey, even if this friend is not in the weight class. If you have someone on your side and not alone, it makes it much easier for you to stay on track. Tell your family that you are on a diet so that it does not help you add the mashed potato. (Mom is famous for doing such things!)

**9. Use the computer** - make some conscious decisions and use the score computer to find out exactly how many points a thing is and not just guess. Knowing a few things from other things helps you if you think you are still hungry and want to make another decision.

**10. Exercise** - If you want to shed pounds faster, this is one of the most important things to do. I know it's coming out, and it's tough. But if you have thought and want to lose weight, this is the best thing for your body and health! It not only helps you lose weight but also burns fat, builds some muscle, and even a little extra because you gain a few extra points if you exercise. These are called Activity Points and can be added to your daily intake. So, the more you exercise, the more points you can get, and the more foods you can eat! Of course, just be smart and don't think you should go home after an hour of exercise and eat whatever you want. All you did was not useless if you did. It may help to consume a little protein for half an hour after exercise. This helps the body's metabolism to function better.

**11. Meetings / Support Groups** - This will help you during your trip. You can share stories with other members and see how they work against you. This is not a race, so don't lose if others win faster than you. You will be sure to talk to everyone at these meetings and give you great ideas on everything from snacks to great restaurants to food. If you do this yourself at home, be part of the conversation, and share your stories.

**12- Weigh-Ins - Weekly weighted average weight**. I know it's hard to know that you only gained 1 kilogram after eating healthy all week and exercising. Don't be discouraged, and stay at it. You might try to change some of what you ate. Or if you have not exercised, get started! But as soon as you get in the groove, you eat better, and you feel healthier, and that pound starts to fall! Believe me!

**13. Diet?** Don't think of yourself as always on a diet. This is a change in lifestyle! This is the way you should eat, and when you learn this, you feel that you don't even have a diet. If you feel like you are on a diet, you are now a failure. And when you know the points just above your head, you don't even feel like it's a diet at all. It has become commonplace.

**14. Just live your life - again, if you feel that your diet will not work**. I know when you start dieting, you look hungry all the time. It will change as you get used to your new lifestyle. It's about choice. Make the right choices for the foods you eat and when you go to a restaurant. Up to you.

**15. The New You** - You are stuck, and it works! Excellent! Keep it and get ready!

# Conclusion

Congratulations on making it to the conclusion of this ***"Weight Watchers Freestyle Cookbook"*** navigation guide and collection of delicious recipes.

Developing healthy eating habits is more accessible and more comfortable than you think. If you get used to eating healthy, you will look and feel better. You will also have more energy and think more clearly. Your immune system will be stronger, so you won't get sick often. Healthy eating habits are your ticket to a healthier body and mind.

If you decide to have healthy eating habits, this will affect your whole life.

Try to be aware of the calories and fat you eat each day. Most people have large amounts of calories and fat every day, without even knowing it.

And, especially, remember that eating garbage leads to more dishes. The problem with eating unhealthy foods is that it makes you eat even unhealthy food. A handful of chips makes you want more. Once you've broken your unhealthy eating cycle, it's easier to maintain your weight loss habits.

I hope you'll find this guide as useful and helpful as I have.

## Thanks, and enjoy it!

CPSIA information can be obtained
at www.ICGtesting.com
Printed in the USA
LVHW051910291120
672964LV00028B/1195